THE HEART FACTOR FOOD PLAN

ALSO BY MARY JOAN OEXMANN:

T.A.G.: A Diabetic Food System

THE
HEART FACTOR
FOOD PLAN

❋

Mary Joan Oexmann, M.S., R.D.

WILLIAM MORROW AND COMPANY, INC.
New York

Recognizing the importance of preserving what has been written, it is the policy of William Morrow and Company, Inc., and its imprints and affiliates to have the books it publishes printed on acid-free paper, and we exert our best efforts to that end.

Library of Congress Cataloging-in-Publication Data

Oexmann, Mary Joan.
    The heart factor food plan / Mary Joan Oexmann.
        p.   cm.
    ISBN 0-688-08848-1
    1. Heart—Diseases—Diet therapy.   2. Heart—Diseases—Nutritional
aspects.   3. Heart—Diseases—Prevention.   I. Title.
RC684.D5049   1990
616.1'205—dc20   89-27721
                                                                          CIP

Printed in the United States of America

First Edition

1 2 3 4 5 6 7 8 9 10

BOOK DESIGN BY HELENE BERINSKY

To my patients

Preface

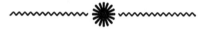

Most of my patients have high blood pressure, coronary artery disease, diabetes, obesity, or some combination of these medical problems. All of my patients can benefit from the advice and information in this book. The health questions that they most frequently ask me—about sodium, cholesterol, fiber, vitamins and minerals, and exercise—are answered here. This book provides sound, sensible, practical nutritional information; it also gives the medical and scientific backgrounds for its recommendations, and motherly advice. The author has a master's degree in nutrition, and years of experience in nutritional clinical research and dietary counseling of patients with obesity, diabetes, high blood pressure, and heart disease.

We live in a time of increased awareness of food and its relationship to health. It is also a time of fad diets and talk-show segments devoted to their proponents. Weight-loss centers and marketing of their associated products constitute a multimillion-dollar-a-year enterprise. Many diet books, weight-loss programs, and low-calorie foods are based on good nutritional principles, but some have no scientific basis, contradict proven medical and nutritional advice; and, in rare circumstances, may be dangerous to health. All of these diet books, weight-loss centers, and special foods (and their cost) can be replaced by a single source of sound information and normal foods.

Unlike many fad diets, this book does not promise something for nothing. Calories do count! The only way to lose weight is to reduce caloric intake or increase the number of calories expended. There is no magic formula or special food that will do the trick. Any effective diet reduces caloric intake at the same time that the special foods are ingested or special regimens are employed. A sensible, practical approach is necessary in order to lose weight.

Most dieters view weight loss as a war. One example is the use of the term "battle of the bulge." In a war, nobody wins. If a dieter approaches weight loss as a war, he or she may experience a temporary decrease in weight, but in the long run it is the rare person with this mindset who loses weight and keeps it off. Fortunately, the process of losing weight and maintaining a healthy diet does not have to be a war. There are practical, relatively painless changes in life-style that can lead to long-term reduction to ideal weight and to improved health.

This book can be used in several ways. For the compulsive and mathematically inclined, there are formulas for calculating daily energy expenditure and tables providing information on the caloric expenditure involved in various activities, the nutrient contents of meals, and the percentage increase in risk of heart disease as a result of excess weight, high blood pressure, high cholesterol, and smoking. For less compulsive or less mathematically oriented readers, there are practical, easy-to-use tables and advice. Even without the use of calculations or tables, it is easy to profit from this book. For example, taking simple measures, such as having one less alcoholic drink per day, not having cream in coffee, or taking a brisk thirty-minute daily walk can result in a weight loss of eight to fifteen pounds of fat a year.

The Heart Factor Food Plan has no glitz or glamour. It is unlikely to result in an appearance by the author on the Phil Donahue or Johnny Carson show. It does not promote an expensive line of diet foods. However, this book has been a help to me, it will benefit my patients, and it can help to improve the health of all who read it.

Timothy C. Fagan, M.D., F.A.C.P.
Director, Hypertension Clinic
Associate Professor of Internal Medicine and Pharmacology
Arizona Health Sciences Center,
Tucson, Arizona

Acknowledgments

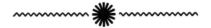

Our current understanding of food decisions for health is a result of years of research by many. For example, the Framingham Heart Study was an eighteen-year study involving over five thousand volunteers. Dr. Thomas Royle Dawber coordinated this monumental effort, which has led to our appreciation of the risk factors of heart and blood vessel disease.

The entire staff of the General Clinical Research Center, in Charleston, South Carolina, has been very supportive of the writing of *The Heart Factor Food Plan.* Advancements in medical science are made through the sum of individual efforts of the clinical investigators, dietary staff, nursing staff, laboratory staff, and volunteers.

It has been my privilege to work with the entire staff of the Medical University of South Carolina Hypertension Clinic. They have contributed to the care of many people. As a team, they stress the importance of compliance with medications and healthful life-style changes based on the needs of the individual.

My appreciation goes to Dr. Timothy C. Fagan, Director

of the Hypertension Clinic, Arizona Health Sciences Center, for his writing of the Preface.

Bill Adler, my agent, has encouraged my writing by identifying William Morrow and Company, Inc., as an excellent publisher. My gratitude goes to Randy Ladenheim-Gil, editor, and her assistant, Christie Neill. The talents of Sonia Greenbaum, copy editor, are greatly appreciated. She always knew what I was trying to say.

My husband, Jack Pickett, understood when I needed to write. He also knows how to cook a good meal when I don't want to make any more food decisions. My cat, Lucifer, continues to remind me that I don't have to be a Type A person to be happy.

The American Heart Association has contributed by supporting research and making information available to all.

Contents

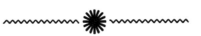

Introduction

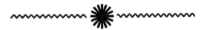

This book was composed during the pleasurable activity of walking. Because of my English heritage, walking has always been a natural. It is a time to organize my thoughts without interruption. It is just a coincidence that there are health benefits to walking. My weight used to be 125 pounds. It still is. Sorry, no testimony about losing 100 pounds in six months and keeping it off for ten years.

The Heart Factor Food Plan is for those who are at risk of being one of the million people who die each year in the United States from heart and blood vessel disease. It gives you an opportunity to improve your health and happiness by making a long-term commitment to selecting foods for health.

This book will help if you are overweight, have heart disease or high blood pressure, or simply want to learn more about nutrition and health. Food and exercise complement your total health care plan. However, food decisions for health are not a substitute for having your blood pressure checked and taking the medicines your doctor may prescribe.

Nutrition is the study of the food chain, from food production to final nutrient utilization by the body. Foods are unique, complex mixtures of many nutrients. Therefore, tables emphasizing the nutrients related to the heart are provided to help you make food decisions. Numerous examples comparing foods illustrate the power of simple food modifications.

It is my personal goal to provide motivation through providing information to people who need food solutions to attain health. The information presented is based on fifteen years of helping people make food decisions. *The Heart Factor Food Plan* is for those who continue to make nutrition interesting and a challenge.

How Many People?

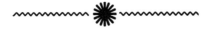

Our newspapers are filled with reports of death caused by automobile accidents, homicide, and suicide. In the United States sixteen people die every hour from these violent causes. Cancer is a devastating illness that may attack the skin, lungs, digestive system, reproductive system, blood, or any part of the body. Every hour of every day, fifty-three people die from cancer.

Almost one million people die each year in the United States from heart and blood vessel disease. This is equal to the combined populations of Washington, D.C., and Miami, Florida. It equals the combined populations of Atlanta, Georgia, and Denver, Colorado. Every hour of every day, 110 people die from cardiovascular disease!

This year 1.5 million Americans will have a heart attack and about 540,000 of them will die. Three hundred thousand people will die before reaching a hospital. One fifth of them will be younger than age sixty-five.

Mortality in the United States

	1970	1980	1985	1987
Total Number	1,921,000	1,989,800	2,086,400	2,125,100
Cardiovascular	1,008,000	988,500	977,900	962,400
Heart disease	735,500	761,100	771,200	759,400
Stroke	207,200	170,200	153,100	148,700
Atherosclerosis	31,700	29,400	23,900	23,100
Other	25,300	27,800	29,700	31,200
Cancer	330,700	416,500	461,600	476,700

Cardiovascular disease kills men and women of all races and all ages through heart attacks and strokes. The National Center for Health Statistics tracks mortality statistics in addition to the number of people with chronic health problems that lead to their increased risk to cardiovascular disease. Approximately fifty-eight million Americans have high blood pressure. Thirty-nine million Americans under the age of sixty-five have heart conditions. In the war against this unnecessary loss in both length and quality of life, making food decisions for health can be one of your strongest weapons!

The statistics are disturbing when I think of the two thousand people in our own high blood pressure clinic. Through the years I have met and cared for many wonderful people. I don't want to face the fact that many will die from a heart attack or stroke.

People may sometimes choose to keep their heads in the sand. They like to keep the youthful belief that "it won't happen to me." If I had high blood pressure, I would probably try to deny it. However, I hope that a health care provider would take the time to point out the risks and the power of change in life-style. I would want the health care provider to help me set priorities. Change is hard, but I would want to know clearly what changes would have the greatest benefit to my health.

The incidence of hypertension and heart conditions increases with age. Only 2 percent of people under the age of eighteen, compared to 43 percent of people between the ages of sixty-five and seventy-five, have high blood pressure.

Incidence of Chronic Health Problems by Age

Age	Heart Condition	Hypertension	Diabetes
<18 years	2.1 %	2.3 %	0.2 %
18–44 years	4.0 %	6.4 %	0.9 %
45–64 years	12.9 %	25.9 %	5.2 %
65–74 years	27.7 %	42.7 %	10.9 %
75+ years	34.9 %	39.5 %	9.6 %

Cardiovascular disease costs every man, woman, and child about $350 each year. The estimated total expenditure on cardiovascular disease in 1988 was $83.7 billion. This figure can be itemized as follows:

Hospital and nursing home services	$53.7 billion
Lost output due to disability	$14.6 billion
Physician and nursing services	$11.3 billion
Medications	$ 4.1 billion
TOTAL:	$83.7 billion

My hope is that the fifty-eight million people living in the United States who have hypertension will incorporate smart food decisions and exercise into their daily lives. It is my hope also that they will encourage their loved ones to do likewise. It represents a commitment to increase one's life expectancy through improvement in the quality of life.

The figures used in this chapter come from the National Center for Health Statistics, U.S. Department of Health and Human Services, and from the American Heart Association, Dallas, Texas. Both resources monitor the trends on an annual basis.

Blood Pressure and the Heart

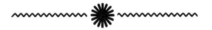

The heart pumps blood through blood vessels to supply essential nutrients to all cells. Blood contains the nutrients of water, protein, carbohydrate, fat, minerals, and vitamins. All cells must have nutrition to live.

Think about glue in a squeeze bottle. Take off the cap, squeeze the container, and out comes the glue. You use the muscle in your hand to apply pressure to force the glue out of the container. Your heart is a muscle that applies pressure to force the blood out of the heart, into the blood vessels, and back to the heart.

The greatest amount of pressure against the walls of the blood vessels occurs when the heart contracts. This force is known as the systolic blood pressure. A lower amount of pressure against the walls of the blood vessels occurs when the heart relaxes and blood is filling the heart. This force is known as the diastolic blood pressure. There are normal fluctuations in blood pressure that occur from moment to moment as you change activity. Your blood pressure decreases when you are at rest or sleeping and increases when you are active.

Drugstores frequently have machines to measure your blood pressure. These machines should only serve as a reminder to have your blood pressure checked. Rely on your doctor or other medical professionals to determine what your blood pressure is and should be.

If your blood pressure is consistently elevated, the diagnosis of "secondary" or "essential" hypertension will be made. Your doctor will do tests to determine if the elevation in blood pressure is secondary to a specific abnormality in the body. If the hypertension cannot be traced to a specific abnormality in the body, the diagnosis of "essential hypertension" will be made. Approximately 90 percent of the population with high blood pressure has essential hypertension. Treatment consists of reducing the risk factors of cardiovascular disease. This may include medications to reduce the blood pressure, life-style changes in diet and exercise, and not smoking.

The American Heart Association has called high blood pressure "the silent killer." Without warning, uncontrolled hypertension may lead to a heart attack or stroke. Death may be the first symptom.

There are a number of factors that increase blood pressure. Fat deposits along the walls of blood vessels narrow the openings through which the blood flows. The heart must work harder to force the blood through narrowed blood vessels. Once again, think of the squeeze bottle of glue. If you are careless about replacing the cap, the glue will dry and harden to narrow the opening. You must apply much more pressure to force the glue out of the smaller opening.

The amount of blood in your body increases as your weight increases. A fifty-year-old man weighing 160 pounds has a blood volume of 5.1 liters. The same man weighing 220 pounds has a blood volume of 6.3 liters. The heart must work harder or increase in size to adapt to the increased demand.

Recognizing the incidence and risk for having a heart

attack or stroke, you may be seriously motivated to wonder about what you can do about it. There are alternative food decisions you can make that may greatly decrease your risk for having diabetes, hypertension, heart disease, a heart attack or stroke. Many people who have survived a heart attack or stroke have gone on to enjoy a productive life by making lifetime changes in diet and exercise, and by not smoking.

Assess your heart and blood vessel system by having your blood pressure checked by a professional. Don't be discouraged. You can take real steps to improve your health. Do it for yourself and your family.

The "Diet Sheet"

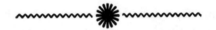

"**M**y doctor tells me that if I lose thirty pounds I may be able to decrease my blood pressure and cholesterol. If I knock off the weight, I won't have to take additional medicine. Just give my wife one of those 'diet sheets' and tell her what to do. My dad died of a heart attack when he was fifty years old. I am forty-five years old. I will do whatever you say."

Many messages are expressed in this monologue. This person knows that high blood pressure and heart disease are serious. This person does not want to take more medicine. Also, this person wants to shift the responsibility of losing thirty pounds to the nutritionist, who will then shift it to his wife. What would you do if you were the nutritionist?

What does the word "diet" mean to you? Does it mean doing without? Are foods either "good" or "bad"? Perhaps diet means starvation and grapefruit. To me that sounds pretty boring, and I like grapefruit. Food decisions do not have to be equivalent to suffering. Diet does not have to be a four-letter word!

Food is a complex mixture of many nutrients. Therefore,

22

there are many food combinations that will satisfy your nutrient goals and your palate. For success, food selection and meal pattern must be acceptable to you. Designing the diet is a series of negotiations that match nutrient composition with your individual preferences and requirements.

While it would be foolish to write a book on making food decisions for health without providing a sample food pattern, keep in mind that this chapter was written to help you get that "quick fix" on food selection. I hope that by the time you finish reading and studying this book, you will have the confidence to make food decisions based on knowing your nutrient goals, food composition, and the power of change.

Diet refers simply to foods and beverages you regularly consume. It is a fact of life. You have to eat to live. My patients are frequently surprised by how I work into their diets the foods they have already decided are forbidden. Guilt is not an essential nutrient! I know that I would comply with "absolutely not" for about twelve minutes. Eating Mom's homemade pumpkin pie on Thanksgiving Day can't be "bad." The challenge is to figure out how to eat a large variety of foods without compromising your long-term nutritional goals.

The "diet sheet" does not have magical powers. Perhaps it can be a guide or reminder if taped to the refrigerator, bathroom scales, and kitchen cabinet. I also know that most "diet sheets" collect dust and add little to your understanding of the relationship between what you eat and health. Changing a lifetime of food decisions is truly more complicated than a simple "diet sheet." Eating smart is a long-term commitment to staying informed about food and how it relates to your health.

With that introduction, here is a "diet sheet" that includes information about foods, amounts, and times of day. The reasons for selecting these foods and times of day are numerous. There are many alternative low-fat food combinations that lead to success. There is no doubt in my mind that if you follow the "diet sheet," you will lose weight.

BREAKFAST

1 cup shredded-wheat cereal
1 cup skim milk
1 banana

LUNCH

1½ cups garden salad
(combination of lettuce, tomatoes, squash,
mushrooms, bell peppers, and cucumbers)
½ cup low-fat cottage cheese, or
½ cup water-packed tuna
iced tea or diet soda

AFTERNOON SNACK

orange, tangerine, or apple

SUPPER

4 ounces chicken or fish
½ cup peas, corn, rice, or potatoes
1 cup broccoli, green beans, cabbage, or spinach
sugarless beverage

EVENING SNACK

peach, pear, or pineapple

The timing of food or food pattern is very important for long-term success. Imitate those who have achieved normal weight for health. Many overweight people skip breakfast and overeat later. This leads to poor portion-size skills. Discipline is required as you form new habits of smart food portions. Similar to a language, these habits are learned.

Food preparation time is frequently given as an excuse for skipping breakfast. It takes thirty seconds to prepare shredded wheat, milk, and a banana. Shredded wheat is preportioned, contains no sugar or added salt, and is high in fiber.

As you develop portioning skills, some reasonable substitutions for shredded wheat are bran flakes, Fiber One, Grapenuts, Chex cereals, Cream of Wheat, and oatmeal. Most people do not use a full cup of milk with cereal. The extra milk can be used in coffee or tea throughout the day.

Skim milk is preferred as it provides essential protein and calcium without added fat or extra calories. However, I do believe in negotiation. Use six ounces of 2 percent fat milk instead of eight ounces of skim milk with the understanding that long-term goals are met. The banana is high in fiber and potassium. Have a whole instead of a half banana. Food should be attractive, nutritious, and appealing. The thought of a brown leftover half banana is not very appealing.

A garden salad at lunch can be varied to prevent boredom. Any combination of lettuce, tomato, bell pepper, celery, squash, cucumber, mushrooms, etc., can be used. All these foods are available at standard salad bars. Salads can be crunchy. Salads do not have to be saturated with fatty dressings that take out the crunch and make a salad slide down. Crunchy salads take more time to eat and to clean your teeth. Parsley, chives, radish, onion, and vinegar add a little zing. Consult the spice chart in the recipe chapter for additional flavoring ideas. Dressings that do not contain oil are alternatives. Low-fat cottage cheese, water-packed tuna, or chicken are all convenient sources of protein. During the winter, you might like homemade soup rather than a salad.

A fresh-fruit snack in the afternoon and evening helps you avoid a large evening meal. Juice is all right, but it is consumed in a third of the time it takes to eat fresh fruit. Fresh fruit is conveniently preportioned. Also, the skin provides nutrients and fiber not found in juice. Fruit with its natural sweetness decreases the sugar habit.

The evening meal is the sensible kind your mother would fix. It provides a lean meat, a starch, and a vegetable. Do not add fat or sugar during food preparation. If you are in the habit of eating one meal a day, this meal will represent the greatest change. Frequently, people ask if it's all right to skip meals and have the larger meal later. Eating only one large meal does not promote good portion sense. Also, skipping meals will lead to being so hungry at mealtimes that you will want to eat the meal, the refrigerator, and the kitchen sink.

This diet contains approximately 1,000 calories. Compliance will result in significant weight loss over time. Food preparation is critical, as it is easy to double calories by using fats and sugar while keeping the amount of food the same.

Structuring a food pattern for life involves a series of negotiations. Change is the first essential ingredient. Foods are not "good" or "bad." Food portion, food preparation, and frequency are much more important than individual foods. All foods can be incorporated into your diet today by using a walking and food-exchange system. This can be found in the chapter on exercise. Determine the distance you have to walk to consume numerous foods without risking weight gain or feeling guilty!

For example, to add one glazed doughnut to the basic diet, you need to walk 1½ miles. You can walk, jog, run, or skip. Extra portions require additional walking. Part of the education process is to learn to include more foods while you safely reach your health goal. Don't spend money until it is in the bank. Have the desired food or beverage after you have completed your walk.

Diet does not have to be a four-letter word!

Risk Factors:
The Power of Change

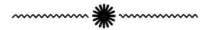

The Framingham Heart Study was conducted from 1949–1967 by Dr. Thomas Royle Dawber and many other scientists in Framingham, Massachusetts. More than five thousand men and women who initially did not have any sign of heart or blood vessel disease volunteered for the study. A health assessment of these people was done every two years for a total of eighteen years. Through this large and long-term study, "risk factors" were identified as being associated with heart and blood vessel disease.

Setting priorities in making life-style decisions requires a thoughtful health assessment. How do your chances of being one of the victims of heart and blood vessel disease compare to those of other people? How do you measure up in terms of the risk factors? What can you do to improve your odds?

You don't have to be a mathematician to understand odds or probability. What is the probability of winning a game of bingo when ten people play? Since there is only one winner, your chance of winning is one winner divided by ten players. The probability of winning is one in ten. This equals a

10 percent chance. What is the probability of winning a game of bingo when one hundred people play? The probability of winning is one in one hundred, or a 1 percent chance. The probability of winning a state lottery is very, very low because thousands of people play the lottery.

What has this got to do with heart and blood vessel disease? What are your chances for developing heart and blood vessel disease? In this chapter you will learn the odds. You will understand the relative importance of each risk factor. The numbers are derived from the Framingham study. For comparison, we will look at the relationship of blood cholesterol and blood pressure on the probability of developing coronary artery disease within eight years in forty-five-year-old men who do not smoke. The figures have been rounded off to simplify the math.

Chance for Developing Heart and Blood Vessel Disease
45-Year-Old Man, Nonsmoker

Sys.BP*	Cholesterol (mg/dl)						
	185	210	235	260	285	310	335
105	2%	3%	3%	4%	6%	7%	9%
120	2%	3%	4%	5%	7%	8%	11%
135	3%	4%	5%	6%	8%	10%	12%
150	3%	4%	6%	7%	9%	12%	15%
165	4%	5%	7%	8%	11%	14%	17%
180	5%	6%	8%	10%	13%	16%	19%
195	6%	7%	9%	12%	15%	18%	22%

*Systolic blood pressure (mmHg)

A forty-five-year-old man who has a blood cholesterol of 235 mg/dl and a systolic blood pressure of 150 mmHg has a 6 percent chance of developing heart and blood vessel disease within eight years. Reading the table the way you read a mileage table on maps, match the blood cholesterol number at the top with the systolic blood pressure number listed on the left to find the probability of developing heart and blood vessel disease. A 6 percent chance is equal to winning at bingo if you were playing with seventeen people.

Each risk factor will be evaluated by comparing the 6 percent risk with a new probability that occurs when each risk factor is taken into account. Setting priorities is simplified by focusing on changes that have the greatest health benefit. This is called perspective.

Perform a personal health assessment by answering the following questions. There are two kinds of risk factors. First, there are the factors that you can't do much about, such as age, gender, and a positive family history for heart disease. Second, there are risk factors that you can do something about. You will be able to identify the power of improving your odds by decreasing risk factors.

Do not be alarmed if you answer "yes" to many of these questions. You are not alone!

Age. Are you older than forty-five?

The frequency of high blood pressure and heart conditions greatly increases with age. This is consistent for both men and women. You cannot do much about your age, which is why it is so important to work on the factors that you can do something about.

Age	Heart Condition	Hypertension
<18 years	2.1%	2.3%
18–44 years	4.0%	6.4%
45–64 years	12.9%	25.9%
65–74 years	27.7%	42.7%
75+ years	34.9%	39.5%

A sixty-five-year-old man with a cholesterol of 235 mg/dl and a systolic blood pressure of 150 mmHg has a 13 percent chance of developing heart and blood vessel disease versus the 6 percent chance that a forty-five-year-old man has. A 13 percent chance is comparable to winning a game of bingo when only seven people are playing! The sixty-five-year-old man has more than doubled his chances of developing heart disease in eight years as compared to the forty-five-year-old man.

Chance for Developing Heart and Blood Vessel Disease
65-Year-Old Man, Nonsmoker

Sys.BP*	Cholesterol (mg/dl)						
	185	210	235	260	285	310	335
105	7%	7%	8%	8%	9%	10%	10%
120	8%	9%	9%	10%	11%	11%	12%
135	9%	10%	11%	12%	12%	13%	14%
150	11%	12%	13%	14%	15%	15%	16%
165	13%	14%	15%	16%	17%	18%	19%
180	15%	16%	17%	18%	19%	21%	22%
195	17%	19%	20%	21%	22%	24%	25%

*Systolic blood pressure (mmHg)

Gender. Are you a man?

Men are more likely than women to have a heart attack, stroke, and atherosclerosis (hardening of the arteries). This is consistent for all ages up to sixty.

Chance for Developing Heart and Blood Vessel Disease
45-Year-Old Woman, Nonsmoker

Sys.BP*	Cholesterol (mg/dl)						
	185	210	235	260	285	310	335
105	1%	1%	1%	2%	2%	2%	3%
120	1%	1%	2%	2%	2%	3%	3%
135	1%	2%	2%	2%	3%	3%	4%
150	2%	2%	2%	3%	3%	4%	5%
165	2%	2%	3%	3%	4%	5%	6%
180	2%	3%	3%	4%	5%	6%	7%
195	3%	3%	4%	5%	6%	7%	9%

*Systolic blood pressure (mmHg)

A woman who does not smoke and has a systolic blood pressure of 150 mmHg and a blood cholesterol of 235 mg/dl has a 2 percent chance of developing heart and blood vessel disease within eight years. This is equal to winning at bingo with fifty people playing!

Chance for Developing Heart and Blood Vessel Disease

Age	Men	Women	Age	Men	Women
35 years	1.9%	0.6%	55 years	10.4%	5.4%
40 years	3.5%	1.2%	60 years	12.0%	7.0%
45 years	5.6%	2.2%	65 years	12.6%	8.1%
50 years	8.1%	3.7%	70 years	12.0%	8.5%

The ratio of men to women for the incidence of sudden cardiac death is three to one. Sudden cardiac death is defined as one that is unexpected in people with or without a history of preexisting heart disease who die within one to six hours of onset. Many times the victim will have been observed to be well within the preceding twenty-four hours.

Women should not feel overly confident that heart and blood vessel disease won't happen to them. Forty-five percent of women die within the first year after a heart attack as contrasted to 20 percent of men!

Heredity. Have your parents, grandparents, or any of your siblings had atherosclerosis, a heart attack, or a stroke? Have you had a heart attack in the past?

An inherited form of severe hypercholesterolemia (high blood cholesterol) is characterized by heart attacks in each generation. This form of coronary heart disease is rare. It is important to remember that families share life-styles in addition to heredity. You are more likely to overeat, smoke, and be inactive if your parents set those examples.

If you have already had a heart attack, your risk for death from heart and blood vessel disease increases fivefold compared to an individual who has never had a heart attack.

Enlargement of the left ventricle. The heart contains four chambers: the right and left ventricles and the right and left atria. Enlargement of the left ventricle of the heart can be determined by electrocardiogram (EKG). The Framingham Heart Study used this criterion to predict risk for heart muscle disease.

**Chance for Developing Heart and Blood Vessel Disease
45-Year-Old Man with Enlarged Left Ventricle**

	Cholesterol (mg/dl)						
Sys.BP*	185	210	235	260	285	310	335
105	3%	4%	6%	7%	9%	11%	14%
120	4%	5%	7%	8%	11%	13%	17%
135	5%	6%	8%	10%	12%	16%	19%
150	6%	7%	9%	12%	15%	18%	22%
165	7%	8%	11%	14%	17%	21%	25%
180	8%	10%	13%	16%	19%	24%	29%
195	9%	12%	15%	18%	22%	27%	33%

*Systolic blood pressure (mmHg)

A positive history for an enlarged left ventricle (left ventricular hypertrophy—LVH) increases the risk of developing heart and blood vessel disease from 6 to 9 percent in a forty-five-year-old man who does not smoke, has a blood cholesterol of 235 mg/dl, and a systolic blood pressure of 150 mmHg.

In the Framingham Heart Study, 62 percent of the people with an enlarged left ventricle died within ten years.

The combined factors of age, gender, positive family history, and enlargement of the left ventricle greatly increase your risk for developing heart and blood vessel disease. For contrast, consider the risk of a thirty-five-year-old woman who does not have LVH with that of a sixty-five-year-old man who does have LVH.

Chance for Developing Heart and Blood Vessel Disease
35-Year-Old Woman

Sys.BP*	Cholesterol (mg/dl)						
	185	210	235	260	285	310	335
105	0%	0%	0%	0%	1%	1%	1%
120	0%	0%	0%	1%	1%	1%	1%
135	0%	0%	1%	1%	1%	1%	1%
150	0%	0%	1%	1%	1%	1%	2%
165	0%	1%	1%	1%	1%	2%	2%
180	1%	1%	1%	1%	1%	2%	2%
195	1%	1%	1%	1%	2%	2%	3%

*Systolic blood pressure (mmHg)

Chance for Developing Heart and Blood Vessel Disease
65-Year-Old Man with Enlargement of the Left Ventricle

Sys.BP*	Cholesterol (mg/dl)						
	185	210	235	260	285	310	335
105	11%	12%	13%	13%	14%	15%	16%
120	13%	14%	15%	16%	17%	18%	19%
135	15%	16%	17%	18%	19%	20%	22%
150	17%	18%	20%	21%	22%	23%	25%
165	20%	21%	23%	24%	25%	27%	28%
180	23%	24%	26%	27%	29%	30%	32%
195	26%	28%	29%	31%	33%	34%	36%

*Systolic blood pressure (mmHg)

There is a tenfold difference in risk based on factors you cannot do anything about!

Now consider the risk factors that you can do something about. This will help you to set priorities and guide you through the process of recognizing the power of change.

Cholesterol. Is your blood cholesterol greater than 200 mg/dl?

The American Heart Association Pooling Project was a ten-year study of eight thousand men. The study concluded that your chances for having a heart attack increase fourfold as your blood cholesterol increases from 175 mg/dl to 300 mg/dl. The higher the cholesterol, the higher the risk.

Consider the example shown below, taken from the Framingham Heart Study. If a systolic blood pressure is constant at 150 mmHg, the risk for developing heart and blood vessel disease increases from 3 percent to 15 percent (a fivefold increase) when blood cholesterol changes from 185 mg/dl to 335 mg/dl. A 15 percent risk is comparable to playing bingo with seven people!

Chance for Developing Heart and Blood Vessel Disease
45-Year-Old Man, Nonsmoker

Sys.BP*	Cholesterol (mg/dl)						
	185	210	235	260	285	310	335
105	2%	3%	3%	4%	6%	7%	9%
120	2%	3%	4%	5%	7%	8%	11%
135	3%	4%	5%	6%	8%	10%	12%
150	3%	4%	6%	7%	9%	12%	15%
165	4%	5%	7%	8%	11%	14%	17%
180	5%	6%	8%	10%	13%	16%	19%
195	6%	7%	9%	12%	15%	18%	22%

*Systolic blood pressure (mmHg)

Blood pressure. Is your systolic blood pressure greater than 140 mmHg?

If blood cholesterol is constant at 235 mg/dl, the risk for developing heart and blood vessel disease increases from 3 percent to 9 percent when systolic blood pressure changes from 105 mmHg to 195 mmHg. There is a threefold increase in risk when blood pressure increases.

Twenty-five million Americans are estimated to have essential hypertension. Ten percent of the American population has a systolic blood pressure greater than 155 mmHg. Successful weight reduction may decrease the incidence of hypertension by 40 percent!

Smoking. Do you smoke?

In *Merchants of Death* by Larry C. White, published in 1988, the author does an excellent job of detailing the impact of tobacco products on our society. Two billion dollars per year are spent on advertising cigarettes. Six hundred billion cigarettes are sold each year to support this addiction. More than 360,000 people die each year as a result of smoking! The relationship between cigarette smoking and cardiovascular disease is significant. This tragic loss may change if young people learn to not start smoking.

Percent of Population that Smokes

	White Men	Black Men	White Women	Black Women
1965	52.4 %	59.6 %	34.1 %	32.7 %
1986	29.5 %	32.5 %	23.7 %	25.1 %

Smoking habits are changing. Unfortunately, women are not getting the message. More women die from lung cancer than breast cancer.

Chance for Developing Heart and Blood Vessel Disease
45-Year-Old Man, Smoker

Sys.BP*	Cholesterol (mg/dl)						
	185	210	235	260	285	310	335
105	3%	4%	5%	7%	8%	11%	13%
120	4%	5%	6%	8%	10%	12%	16%
135	4%	6%	7%	9%	12%	15%	18%
150	5%	7%	9%	11%	14%	17%	21%
165	6%	8%	10%	13%	16%	19%	24%
180	7%	9%	12%	15%	18%	22%	27%
195	9%	11%	14%	17%	21%	26%	31%

*Systolic blood pressure (mmHg)

The forty-five-year-old man who has a blood cholesterol of 235 mg/dl and a systolic blood pressure of 150 mmHg increases his risk for developing heart and blood vessel disease from 6 percent to 9 percent when he starts smoking. The risk increases as the amount of smoking increases.

Increase in Risk Due to Smoking—Men

Age Range	Less Than 1 Pack	1 Pack	More Than 1 Pack
45–54 years	29%	67%	115%
55–64 years	15%	32%	51%
65–74 years	12%	24%	39%

Tobacco smoke contains carbon monoxide, which displaces oxygen from hemoglobin circulating in the blood. The heart has to work harder to retain oxygen in the blood. Carbon monoxide may also damage the walls of the arteries. The arteries become more vulnerable to fat deposits that help narrow the walls. Also, smoking increases your chances for developing heart-rhythm disturbances, which may lead to sudden death.

If you are thirty to thirty-five years old and smoke two packs of cigarettes each day, you have a reduced life expectancy of eight to nine years. A man aged forty-five to fifty-four who smokes two packs of cigarettes each day doubles his risk of developing heart and blood vessel disease. However, the risk of dying from coronary heart disease is ten times greater than for a person who does not smoke. Ten percent of the American population smokes one or more packs of cigarettes a day.

In 1975 the death toll due to smoking was 266,000. The causes of death are: 160,000 from coronary heart disease, 64,000 from lung cancer, 20,000 from cancers at other sites, and 22,000 from chronic lung disease. The shocking fact is that this loss to society is self-inflicted. It is preventable!

It is hard to change smoking habits because smoking is addictive. Sometimes people gain weight after kicking the habit. If it comes down to either gaining five or ten pounds or kicking the habit, please quit smoking! It will have the greatest health benefit.

Glucose tolerance. Do you have high blood sugar?

People who have high blood sugar caused by diabetes have an increased risk to developing heart and blood vessel disease. The risk changes from 6 percent to 7 percent when systolic blood pressure is 150 mmHg and blood cholesterol is 235 mg/dl.

**Chance for Developing Heart and Blood Vessel Disease
45-Year-Old Man, Abnormal Glucose Tolerance**

	Cholesterol (mg/dl)						
Sys.BP*	185	210	235	260	285	310	335
105	3%	3%	4%	5%	7%	9%	11%
120	3%	4%	5%	6%	8%	10%	13%
135	4%	5%	6%	8%	10%	12%	15%
150	4%	6%	7%	9%	11%	14%	18%
165	5%	7%	8%	10%	13%	16%	20%
180	6%	8%	10%	12%	15%	19%	23%
195	7%	9%	11%	14%	18%	22%	27%

*Systolic blood pressure (mmHg)

Ninety percent of people who have diabetes have Type II, or adult-onset diabetes. This type of diabetes usually occurs later in life. Insulin replacement may not be required. Weight reduction is frequently the best treatment for normalizing blood sugar.

Body Mass Index (BMI). Is your BMI greater than 26?

Determine your body mass index (BMI) by using the table on pages 40–41. Height is listed at the top. Slide your finger down the column to find your weight in pounds. Your weight will correspond to the BMI listed on the left. For example, if you are five feet six inches and weigh 161 pounds, your BMI is 26. If you are five feet two inches and weigh 162 pounds, your BMI is 30.

For optimal health, your BMI should be about 20. A person between the ages of twenty to forty-four whose BMI is greater than 26 has a 5.6 times greater chance of having diabetes and high blood pressure than a person with a BMI of 20. If your BMI is greater than 36, you have doubled your chance of dying from heart disease.

Body Mass Index

BMI	4'10"	4'11"	5'0"	5'1"	5'2"	5'3"	5'4"	5'5"	5'6"
18	86	89	91	95	97	101	105	108	112
19	90	94	97	100	103	107	111	114	118
20	95	99	102	106	108	113	117	120	124
21	100	104	107	111	114	118	123	126	130
22	105	109	112	116	119	124	129	132	136
23	109	114	117	F121	F124	F130	F135	F138	F143
24	F114	F119	F122	127	130	135	140	M144	M149
25	119	124	127	M132	M135	M141	M146	150	155
26	124	129	132	137	141	146	152	156	161
27	128	134	137	143	146	152	158	162	168
28	133	139	142	148	152	158	164	168	174
29	138	144	147	153	157	163	170	174	180
30	143	149	152	158	162	169	176	180	186
31	147	153	158	164	168	175	181	186	192
32	152	158	163	169	173	180	187	191	199
33	157	163	168	174	179	186	193	197	205
34	162	168	173	180	184	191	199	203	211
35	166	173	178	185	189	197	205	209	217
36	**171**	**178**	**183**	**190**	**195**	**203**	**211**	**215**	**223**
37	176	183	188	195	200	208	217	221	230
38	181	188	193	201	206	214	222	227	236
39	185	193	198	206	211	220	228	233	242
40	190	198	203	211	216	225	234	239	248
41	195	203	208	216	222	231	240	245	254
42	200	208	213	222	227	237	246	251	261
43	204	213	219	227	233	242	252	257	267
44	209	218	224	232	238	248	257	263	273
45	214	223	229	238	244	253	263	269	279
46	219	228	234	243	249	259	269	275	285
47	223	233	239	248	254	265	275	281	292
48	228	238	244	253	260	270	281	287	298
49	233	243	249	259	265	276	287	293	304
50	238	248	254	264	271	282	293	299	310
51	242	252	259	269	276	287	298	305	316
52	247	257	264	275	281	293	304	311	323
53	252	262	269	280	287	298	310	317	329
54	257	267	274	285	292	304	316	323	335
55	261	272	280	290	298	310	322	329	341
56	266	277	285	296	303	315	328	335	347

Optimal BMI is highlighted (F = female; M = male). The risk of dying from heart disease doubles when BMI is greater than 36!

Body Mass Index

BMI	5'7"	5'8"	5'9"	5'10"	5'11"	6'0"	6'1"	6'2"	6'3"
18	114	118	121	126	128	133	135	140	145
19	121	125	128	133	135	140	143	148	153
20	127	132	135	139	143	147	150	155	161
21	134	138	141	146	150	155	158	163	169
22	140	F145	F148	F153	F157	162	166	M171	M177
23	F146	M151	M155	M160	M164	M170	M173	179	185
24	M153	158	162	167	171	177	181	186	193
25	159	164	168	174	178	184	188	194	201
26	165	171	175	181	185	192	196	202	209
27	172	178	182	188	192	199	203	210	217
28	178	184	188	195	200	206	211	217	225
29	184	191	195	202	207	214	218	225	233
30	191	197	202	209	214	221	226	233	241
31	197	204	209	216	221	228	233	241	249
32	203	210	215	223	228	236	241	249	257
33	210	217	222	230	235	243	248	256	265
34	216	224	229	237	242	251	256	264	273
35	223	230	236	244	249	258	263	272	281
36	229	237	242	251	257	265	271	280	289
37	235	243	249	258	264	273	278	287	297
38	242	250	256	265	271	280	286	295	305
39	248	257	263	272	278	287	293	303	313
40	254	263	269	279	285	295	301	311	321
41	261	270	276	286	292	302	308	318	329
42	267	276	283	293	299	310	316	326	337
43	273	283	289	300	307	317	324	334	345
44	280	289	296	307	314	324	331	342	353
45	286	296	303	314	321	332	339	349	361
46	292	303	310	321	328	339	346	357	369
47	299	309	316	328	335	346	354	365	377
48	305	316	323	335	342	354	361	373	385
49	312	322	330	342	349	361	369	381	393
50	318	329	337	349	356	369	376	388	402
51	324	335	343	356	364	376	384	396	410
52	331	342	350	363	371	383	391	404	418
53	337	349	357	370	378	391	399	412	426
54	343	355	364	377	385	398	406	419	434
55	350	362	370	384	392	405	414	427	442
56	356	368	377	391	399	413	421	435	450

Optimal BMI is highlighted (F = female; M = male). The risk of dying from heart disease doubles when BMI is greater than 36!

What is your optimal weight? If you are unsure about your frame size, use the table below to estimate it by measuring your elbow breadth. Extend your arm and bend the forearm upward at a ninety-degree angle. Keep your fingers straight and turn your palm toward your body. Place the thumb and index finger of your other hand on the two prominent bones on either side of your elbow. Measure the space between your fingers against a ruler. If the distance is less than the standard, you have a small frame. If it is greater, you have a large frame.

Height and Elbow Breadth for Men and Women

Height Without Shoes	Elbow Breadth Medium Frame
Men	
5'1"–5'2"	2½"–2⅞"
5'3"–5'6"	2⅝"–2⅞"
5'7"–5'10"	2¾"–3"
5'11"–6'2"	2¾"–3⅛"
6'3"+	2⅞"–3½"
Women	
4'10"–4'11"	2¼"–2½"
4'11"–5'2"	2¼"–2½"
5'3"–5'6"	2⅜"–2⅝"
5'7"–5'10"	2⅜"–2⅝"
5'11"+	2½"–2¾"

Courtesy of the Metropolitan Life Insurance Company

**Desirable Weights for Women, Aged 25 and Older
(in Pounds by Height and Frame; Without Shoes or
Clothing)**

Height	Average	Small	Medium	Large
4'9"	114 lb	99–108	106–118	115–128
4'10"	115 lb	100–110	108–120	117–131
4'11"	117 lb	101–112	110–123	119–134
5'0"	120 lb	103–115	112–126	122–137
5'1"	123 lb	105–118	115–129	125–140
5'2"	125 lb	108–121	118–132	128–144
5'3"	130 lb	111–124	121–135	131–148
5'4"	133 lb	114–127	124–138	134–152
5'5"	137 lb	117–130	127–141	137–156
5'6"	140 lb	120–133	130–144	140–160
5'7"	144 lb	123–136	133–147	143–164
5'8"	147 lb	126–139	136–150	146–167
5'9"	149 lb	129–142	139–153	149–170
5'10"	152 lb	132–145	142–156	152–173
5'11"	155 lb	135–148	145–159	155–176

Courtesy of the Metropolitan Life Insurance Company

Desirable Weights for Men, Aged 25 and Older
(in Pounds by Height and Frame; Without Shoes or
Clothing)

Height	Average	Small	Medium	Large
5'1"	134 lb	123–129	126–136	133–145
5'2"	137 lb	125–131	128–138	135–148
5'3"	139 lb	127–133	130–140	137–151
5'4"	142 lb	129–135	132–143	139–155
5'5"	145 lb	131–137	134–146	141–159
5'6"	148 lb	133–140	137–149	144–163
5'7"	151 lb	135–143	140–152	147–167
5'8"	154 lb	137–146	143–155	150–171
5'9"	157 lb	139–149	146–158	153–175
5'10"	160 lb	141–152	149–161	156–179
5'11"	164 lb	144–155	152–165	159–183
6'0"	167 lb	147–159	155–169	163–187
6'1"	171 lb	150–163	159–173	167–192
6'2"	175 lb	153–167	162–177	171–197
6'3"	180 lb	157–171	166–182	176–202

Courtesy of the Metropolitan Life Insurance Company

Waist-hip ratio (WHR). Assessing your waist-hip ratio (WHR) is a method to characterize the deposition of fat as to region in the body. Men tend to store more fat in the abdominal area compared to women, who store more fat in the legs. People who have a WHR higher than 0.8 are at greater risk of developing heart and blood vessel disease.

What is your WHR? Measure your waist and hips. It can be in inches or centimeters because what you are most interested in is the ratio. If your waist is twenty-five inches and your hips are thirty-six inches, your WHR is 0.7. If your waist is thirty-five inches and your hips are forty inches, your WHR is 0.9.

Exercise. Do you exercise less than three times a week for twenty minutes (one hour total)?

Exercise offers many health benefits. Regular physical activity leads to a reduction in the resting heart rate and blood pressure. However, 60 to 80 percent of the American population is considered physically inactive! Exercise, healthy food decisions, and not smoking are excellent ways to reduce blood pressure and blood cholesterol and to improve glucose tolerance.

Attitude about safety. Do you forget to "buckle up" your seat belt when you travel in a car?

Wearing a seat belt is one way to decrease your risk of bodily harm or even death by an automobile accident. Some states require by law that you buckle up for safety. People who wear seat belts tend to be more likely to take the steps to decrease their risk of having heart and blood vessel disease.

Consider the power of changing risk factors. A forty-five-year-old man who smokes, has an abnormal glucose tolerance, systolic blood pressure of 195 mmHg, and a blood cholesterol of 335 mg/dl has a 36 percent chance of developing heart and blood vessel disease. This is comparable to playing bingo with three people!

Chance for Developing Heart and Blood Vessel Disease
45-Year-Old Man, Smoker with Glucose Intolerance

Sys.BP*	Cholesterol (mg/dl)						
	185	210	235	260	285	310	335
105	4%	5%	6%	8%	10%	13%	16%
120	5%	6%	8%	10%	12%	15%	19%
135	6%	7%	9%	11%	14%	18%	22%
150	7%	8%	10%	13%	16%	20%	25%
165	8%	10%	12%	15%	19%	23%	28%
180	9%	11%	14%	18%	22%	27%	32%
195	11%	13%	17%	20%	25%	30%	36%

*Systolic blood pressure (mmHg)

This same forty-five-year-old man can quit smoking, normalize blood glucose, reduce systolic blood pressure to 120 mmHg, and reduce cholesterol to 185 mg/dl. He would reduce his risk for developing heart and blood vessel disease to 2 percent. This is comparable to playing bingo with fifty people. Change is powerful!

Chance for Developing Heart and Blood Vessel Disease
45-Year-Old Man, Nonsmoker

Sys.BP*	Cholesterol (mg/dl)						
	185	210	235	260	285	310	335
105	2%	3%	3%	4%	6%	7%	9%
120	2%	3%	4%	5%	7%	8%	11%
135	3%	4%	5%	6%	8%	10%	12%
150	3%	4%	6%	7%	9%	12%	15%
165	4%	5%	7%	8%	11%	14%	17%
180	5%	6%	8%	10%	13%	16%	19%
195	6%	7%	9%	12%	15%	18%	22%

*Systolic blood pressure (mmHg)

If you answer "yes" to any of the following questions, you have an increased risk of having or getting heart and blood vessel disease.

Are you older than forty-five?

Have your parents, grandparents, or any of your siblings had a heart attack or stroke? Have you had a heart attack?

Are you a man?

Do you have left ventricular hypertrophy as shown by electrocardiogram?

If you answer "yes" to any of the following questions, you can actively take steps to decrease your risk. Set priorities!

Is your blood cholesterol greater than 200 mg/dl?

Is your systolic blood pressure greater than 140 mmHg?

Do you smoke?

Do you have high blood sugar?

Is your body mass index (BMI) greater than 26?

Is your waist-hip ratio (WHR) greater than 0.8?

Do you exercise less than three times a week for twenty minutes (one hour total)?

Do you forget to "buckle up" your seat belt when you travel in a car?

Favorite Excuses

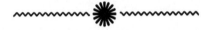

I t's interesting how we talk ourselves into different ways of thinking about nutrition. Excuses are an important part of the process. See if you recognize any of your favorite excuses.

"It's too expensive!" The only time that going on a diet is expensive is when foods are being added to your normal intake instead of being substituted for current food decisions. Eating less food is less expensive. One way to normalize body weight is to reduce the amount of food you currently eat in half. This will cut your food costs in half. While you will probably spend more money on fruits and vegetables, you will easily make up the difference by spending less money on expensive junk food.

"I don't like diet foods." Sensible eating does not require special "diet" foods. Foods for health can be selected from the basic four food groups: fruits and vegetables; dairy products; breads and starches; and meats, poultry, and fish.

* * *

"I'll have to buy new clothes!" I've worn the same size clothes all of my adult life. Since buying clothes in just one size can be expensive, there is no doubt that buying them for multiple sizes can be very expensive. Weight change is usually a gradual process, so you may already have multiple sizes. Invest in clothing that is comfortable. Wear a belt or scarf to accentuate your new waistline. It's much easier to take in a seam than to let it out. Consider your current size and the size that you want to be wearing in two, four, six, and twelve months. Purchase clothing for the long-term goal.

"I lost ten pounds quickly and now the scales won't budge!" As you will learn, part of the initial rapid weight loss is due to a sodium and water loss. It does not reflect a reduction in fat. Also, people rely too much on what the scales say instead of on how they look. It's a good idea to measure your waist and stand on the scales once a week. However, each morning look in the mirror to assess your daily progress. Achieving the long-term goal is the sum of achieving daily goals.

"My spouse loves me the way I am. If I change, he or she won't love me anymore." Your partner does not love you because of your weight but because of your heart and mind. Your partner will be proud of you and your example as you take the steps to improve your health. In most situations your mate will be supportive and enthusiastic. However, do not feel discouraged if your partner seems indifferent. It's a personal decision to select foods for health. Don't force changes onto others.

"I just spent two hundred dollars at the grocery store. I'll begin the diet when I finish the potato chips and cookies." The next food decision begins now. Carefully assess foods that are currently in your kitchen. Are there some that you

could freeze to save for a later time? Ultimately you will be able to include all foods into your meal plan. Focus on making adjustments in preparation and portion size.

"I get so hungry!" Your new food pattern includes eating at specific times throughout the day. Three meals and two snacks are suggested as a starting point. It's comforting to know that there are always less than two or three hours until it's time to eat again. If you get hungry, sip a glass of skim milk or eat a piece of fruit. The foods to avoid are fats and sugar.

"I won't be able to go out to dinner again." Rubbish! Eating out is very much a part of our culture. Participate in this social event while learning to dine smart. Feeling guilty for participating in life leads to resentment and depression. Be your own best friend and eat in a restaurant that offers alternatives to fried foods. Frequently you can order separate salads and share an entree. Ask that dressings or butter be "on the side."

"I'm the only person who has to do this." Over 100 million Americans are trying to lose weight. While it's true that not everyone needs to lose weight, all of us need to make food decisions for health. Achieving long-term nutrition goals is more unique than setting the goal.

"My food will have to be cooked separately from the rest of the family's." The foods you select for your family are from the basic four food groups. They are nutritious and familiar. Your family will appreciate the fact that you value the health of all family members. Fat and portion sizes are reduced for the benefit of all. Cook foods in a single pot!

"I can't exercise. My body aches when I walk." This is a common complaint of people who are constantly carrying extra pounds. Imagine someone handing you a thirty-pound

bag of flour and announcing that you must carry it everywhere. For a few minutes, it's not that big a deal. By the
second hour, it's pretty inconvenient. By the end of the day,
you are really tired. It's not surprising that people who carry
extra weight have more aches and pains. The aches and
pains will decrease as you increase your strength and endur-
ance with exercise. Also, the stress of carrying extra pounds
will decrease as you normalize your weight.

"It hasn't worked before. Why should I bother now?"
Today is the first day of the rest of your life!

"It's hard! It's slow!" Are you spoiled by our "instant"
society? Do you have children who don't want to wait till
Christmas? Consider the things that you have done in your
life that are important. Perhaps you've learned to play a
musical instrument that brings joy to yourself and others.
Achievement requires discipline and a long-term commitment. Safe and successful nutrition takes a lifetime. However, the attitude to achieve nutrition for health can happen
instantly!

"It's a bore!" Making food decisions for health is an interesting challenge to a nutritionist. It's understandable that
most people find it pretty boring. Everyone eats, but not
everyone is a nutritionist. Food decisions for health become
interesting to everyone when they experience the benefits.
To defeat boredom, study some of the many cookbooks
with low-calorie recipes that provide attractive ideas for
new food combinations. Variety helps to decrease boredom.
However, accept that there will be times when it isn't fun.
Stick with your decisions and remember that health benefits
take time.

"I don't want to!" I'm not going to pretend that I can make
food decisions for others. Food decisions for health are a
personal commitment. All I can do is try to help others help

themselves. My hope is to strengthen your motivation through providing information. Your response to the information can be either positive or negative. I hope that you will choose to experience health benefits.

"I'll have to give up social events and my friends." It's ridiculous to associate food decisions for health with giving up your friends! Food decisions for health are positive. Share those decisions with your friends. They will be more understanding than you may think. Don't withdraw from your friends. My hope is that after reading *The Heart Factor Food Plan* you will be thinking about showing off your new figure at the social event you were planning to miss.

"All my family is overweight. I can't change my genes." Families share heredity. Families also share the kitchen, meals, and the refrigerator. This makes it very difficult to know if your weight is the result of heredity, a shared environment, or a combination of the two. However, it becomes irrelevant as change is still the cure. Weight reduction requires calorie reduction.

"I gain five pounds by eating a single food off my diet! I gain two pounds just by thinking about it!" False. Your weight is based on the sum of all food decisions. While foods containing fats are high in calories, a single pat of margarine will have little effect. The decision to chronically consume high-calorie foods leads to weight gain.

"I just have big bones." Funny thing, when I think of a person as being "skin and bones," I think of someone who is very thin. The body is made up of much more than bones. There are specialized tissues that make up many organs. Your goal will be to keep your bones, muscles, and organs healthy while you reduce your total body fat. There aren't many bones in the stomach!

* * *

"My neighbors will think I'm crazy if after twenty years I decide to go for a run!" False. In two weeks some neighbors may be running with you!

"I gave up smoking." There is some debate as to the relationship between decreased smoking and increased body weight. Most likely, you eat more. In any case, the benefits of decreased smoking may be greater than a ten-pound weight gain. The arithmetic remains the same. Weight reduction depends on decreasing calorie intake and/or increasing calorie expenditure.

"It takes too much time!" It takes time to learn about food composition and preparing foods with less fat. Keep meals simple. You are worth the time invested.

"I'm a very busy person. I don't have time to go for a walk!" No doubt President Truman was a very busy person, yet he always made time for his morning walk. When you decide that it is important, you will find the time.

What is your favorite excuse? Think about it. Things can change when you decide to change them! The quality and length of life can be improved. Healthful food decisions are not required by law. It is up to you either to actively make food decisions for health or passively accept ill health.

Calories

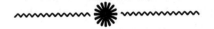

Protein, carbohydrate, fat, and alcohol supply calories for energy. You need calories, units of heat or energy, to live. If you eat more calories (energy) than you need, you will store the excess as fat and gain weight. If you eat fewer calories than you need, your body will supply the needed energy. You will lose weight. The calorie or energy balance over time will determine your weight.

Food is a complex mixture of protein, carbohydrate, fat, water, minerals, and vitamins. Some foods provide greater amounts of individual nutrients and are identified as major food sources.

Protein supplies the body with building blocks for healthy tissue. The building blocks are known as amino acids. Major food sources are dairy products, eggs, meat, and grains. Protein provides four calories per gram. Normal intake is 50 to 80 grams each day. This is equal to 200–320 calories. Protein is made up of carbon, hydrogen, oxygen, and nitrogen. The body breaks down protein into energy, carbon dioxide, water, and ammonia.

Carbohydrate supplies the body with energy. Adequate carbohydrate is important as it protects the protein from being used for energy. When losing weight, you want to be losing fat tissue as opposed to protein-containing tissues such as muscle. Therefore, during weight reduction, consume at least 100 grams of carbohydrate per day. Carbohydrate provides four calories per gram. One hundred grams of carbohydrate provide 400 calories. Major food sources are grains, fruits, vegetables, and milk. Carbohydrate is made up of carbon, hydrogen, and oxygen. The body breaks down carbohydrate into energy, carbon dioxide, and water.

Fat supplies the body with the most concentrated form of energy. When reducing calorie intake, fat is the most important nutrient to modify. Major food sources are butter, margarine, oils, dressings, fatty meats, and whole milk. Fat provides nine calories per gram. On a weight-per-weight basis, fat supplies the body with more than twice the number of calories derived from protein and carbohydrate. During weight reduction, a minimum intake of 30 grams per day is appropriate. This is equal to 270 calories. Fat is made up of carbon, oxygen, and hydrogen. The body breaks down fat into energy, carbon dioxide, and water.

Alcohol provides seven calories per gram. Alcohol contains a different combination of carbon, oxygen, and hydrogen. The body breaks down alcohol into energy, carbon dioxide, and water. There is a positive correlation between high blood pressure and alcohol consumption independent of age, exercise, smoking, and weight. If your weight is normal, do not consume more than one serving of an alcoholic beverage per day. Alcoholic beverages include hard liquor, beer, and wine.

Your calorie requirements increase as your weight increases because it takes more energy to carry the extra weight. Imagine how much more energy you would need to carry fifty pounds of potatoes. It makes me tired to think about it. Consider the calorie requirements of a forty-year-old, five-feet four-inch woman who has a medium activity level. Her energy requirement is 1,660 calories when she weighs 133 pounds and 1,860 calories when she weighs 173 pounds!

Weight and Calorie Requirements
Women, 40 Years Old, 5'4"

		Activity		
% IBW*	Weight	Low	Medium	High
90%	120 lb	1450	1590	1720
100%	133 lb	1520	1660	1790
110%	146 lb	1580	1720	1870
120%	160 lb	1650	1800	1950
130%	173 lb	1710	1860	2020
140%	186 lb	1770	1930	2090

*Percent ideal body weight

It's common for people to adapt gradually to the stress of carrying extra pounds by decreasing activity. Walking a single mile becomes difficult. If you are slim, you may be comfortable walking a mile in fourteen minutes. If you are overweight, you may find it difficult to walk a mile in twenty minutes. It's a natural tendency to avoid what is difficult. You can fall into a frustrating cycle. Weight gain leads to decreased activity and decreased activity leads to weight gain!

Energy requirements are based on gender, height, weight, age, and activity level. The calorie requirement to maintain weight is based on the formula for basal energy expenditure (BEE).

The BEE for women equals the sum of 655; 9.6 times the

desirable weight in kilograms; and 1.7 times height in centimeters. The age in years times 4.7 is subtracted from the
sum.

$$\text{BEE (women)} = 655 + (9.6 \times \text{kg}) + (1.7 \times \text{cm}) - (4.7 \times \text{yr})$$

The BEE for men equals the sum of 66; 13.7 times the
desirable weight in kilograms; and 5.0 times the height in
centimeters. The age in years times 6.8 is subtracted from the
sum.

$$\text{BEE (men)} = 66 + (13.7 \times \text{kg}) + (5. \times \text{cm}) - (6.8 \times \text{yr})$$

The basal energy expenditure is adjusted for activity by
multiplying the BEE by 110 percent for low activity, 120
percent for medium activity, and finally 130 percent for high
activity.

One pound of body fat equals 3,500 calories. Therefore,
reduce your calorie requirement by 500 calories each day to
lose one pound each week. To lose two pounds per week,
reduce your calorie requirement by 1,000 calories. However,
do not restrict your calorie intake to less than 1,000 calories
per day, as you must continue to satisfy all nutrient requirements during weight reduction.

What is your calorie requirement? What is your calorie
requirement to lose one pound each week? Review the following tables. Keep your calorie requirement in mind, since
you will need it when you study food composition later on.

Calorie Requirements for Women

Height	Age	To Maintain Weight Activity Level*			To Lose Weight	
		Low	Medium	High	1 Lb/ Week	2 Lb/ Week
4'9"	20	1490	1620	1760	1120	620
	30	1440	1570	1700	1070	570
	40	1390	1510	1640	1010	510
	50	1330	1460	1580	960	460
	60	1280	1400	1520	900	400
	70	1230	1340	1450	840	340
	80	1180	1290	1390	790	290
	90	1130	1230	1330	730	230
	100	1080	1170	1270	670	170
4'10"	20	1500	1640	1770	1140	640
	30	1450	1580	1710	1080	580
	40	1400	1520	1650	1020	520
	50	1350	1470	1590	970	470
	60	1290	1410	1530	910	410
	70	1240	1350	1470	850	350
	80	1190	1300	1410	800	300
	90	1140	1240	1350	740	240
	100	1090	1190	1280	690	190
4'11"	20	1520	1650	1790	1150	650
	30	1460	1600	1730	1100	600
	40	1410	1540	1670	1040	540
	50	1360	1480	1610	980	480
	60	1310	1430	1550	930	430
	70	1260	1370	1490	870	370
	80	1210	1310	1420	810	310
	90	1150	1260	1360	760	260
	100	1100	1200	1300	700	200
5'0"	20	1530	1670	1810	1170	670
	30	1480	1620	1750	1120	620
	40	1430	1560	1690	1060	560

*Low activity = 110% of basal energy expenditure (BEE); medium activity = 120% of basal energy expenditure (BEE); high activity = 130% of basal energy expenditure (BEE); BEE = 655 + (9.6 × kg) + (1.7 × cm) − (4.7 × years)

Calorie Requirements for Women *continued*

Height	Age	To Maintain Weight Activity Level* Low	Medium	High	To Lose Weight 1 Lb/ Week	2 Lb/ Week
	50	1380	1510	1630	1010	510
	60	1330	1450	1570	950	450
	70	1280	1390	1510	890	390
	80	1220	1340	1450	840	340
	90	1170	1280	1390	780	280
	100	1120	1220	1330	720	220
5'1"	20	1560	1700	1840	1200	700
	30	1500	1640	1780	1140	640
	40	1450	1580	1720	1080	580
	50	1400	1530	1650	1030	530
	60	1350	1470	1600	970	470
	70	1300	1410	1530	910	410
	80	1250	1360	1470	860	360
	90	1190	1300	1410	800	300
	100	1140	1250	1350	750	250
5'2"	20	1570	1710	1860	1210	710
	30	1520	1660	1800	1160	660
	40	1470	1600	1730	1100	600
	50	1420	1540	1670	1040	540
	60	1360	1490	1610	990	490
	70	1310	1430	1550	930	430
	80	1260	1370	1490	870	370
	90	1210	1320	1430	820	320
	100	1160	1260	1370	760	260
5'3"	20	1600	1750	1890	1250	750
	30	1550	1690	1830	1190	690
	40	1500	1630	1770	1130	630
	50	1450	1580	1710	1080	580
	60	1390	1520	1650	1020	520
	70	1340	1460	1590	960	460

*Low activity = 110% of basal energy expenditure (BEE); medium activity = 120% of basal energy expenditure (BEE); high activity = 130% of basal energy expenditure (BEE); BEE = 655 + (9.6 × kg) + (1.7 × cm) − (4.7 × years)

Calorie Requirements for Women *continued*

| Height | Age | To Maintain Weight
Activity Level* | | | To Lose Weight | |
		Low	Medium	High	1 Lb/ Week	2 Lb/ Week
	80	1290	1410	1520	910	410
	90	1240	1350	1460	850	350
	100	1190	1290	1400	790	290
5'4"	20	1620	1770	1920	1270	770
	30	1570	1710	1850	1210	710
	40	1520	1660	1790	1160	660
	50	1470	1600	1730	1100	600
	60	1410	1540	1670	1040	540
	70	1360	1490	1610	990	490
	80	1310	1430	1550	930	430
	90	1260	1370	1490	870	370
	100	1210	1320	1430	820	320
5'5"	20	1650	1800	1940	1300	800
	30	1590	1740	1880	1240	740
	40	1540	1680	1820	1180	680
	50	1490	1630	1760	1130	630
	60	1440	1570	1700	1070	570
	70	1390	1510	1640	1010	510
	80	1340	1460	1580	960	460
	90	1280	1400	1520	900	400
	100	1230	1340	1460	840	340
5'6"	20	1670	1820	1970	1320	820
	30	1610	1760	1910	1260	760
	40	1560	1700	1850	1200	700
	50	1510	1650	1780	1150	650
	60	1460	1590	1720	1090	590
	70	1410	1530	1660	1030	530
	80	1350	1480	1600	980	480
	90	1300	1420	1540	920	420
	100	1250	1370	1480	870	370

*Low activity = 110% of basal energy expenditure (BEE); medium activity = 120% of basal energy expenditure (BEE); high activity = 130% of basal energy expenditure (BEE); BEE = 655 + (9.6 × kg) + (1.7 × cm) − (4.7 × years)

Calorie Requirements for Women *continued*

| Height | Age | To Maintain Weight Activity Level* | | | To Lose Weight | |
		Low	Medium	High	1 Lb/ Week	2 Lb/ Week
5'7"	20	1690	1840	2000	1340	840
	30	1640	1790	1940	1290	790
	40	1590	1730	1880	1230	730
	50	1540	1680	1820	1180	680
	60	1480	1620	1750	1120	620
	70	1430	1560	1690	1060	560
	80	1380	1500	1630	1000	500
	90	1330	1450	1570	950	450
	100	1280	1390	1510	890	390
5'8"	20	1710	1870	2020	1370	870
	30	1660	1810	1960	1310	810
	40	1610	1750	1900	1250	750
	50	1560	1700	1840	1200	700
	60	1500	1640	1780	1140	640
	70	1450	1580	1720	1080	580
	80	1400	1530	1650	1030	530
	90	1350	1470	1590	970	470
	100	1300	1410	1530	910	410
5'9"	20	1730	1880	2040	1380	880
	30	1670	1830	1980	1330	830
	40	1620	1770	1920	1270	770
	50	1570	1710	1860	1210	710
	60	1520	1660	1790	1160	660
	70	1470	1600	1730	1100	600
	80	1420	1540	1670	1040	540
	90	1360	1490	1610	990	490
	100	1310	1430	1550	930	430
5'10"	20	1750	1900	2060	1400	900
	30	1700	1850	2000	1350	850
	40	1640	1790	1940	1290	790

*Low activity = 110% of basal energy expenditure (BEE); medium activity = 120% of basal energy expenditure (BEE); high activity = 130% of basal energy expenditure (BEE); BEE = 655 + (9.6 × kg) + (1.7 × cm) − (4.7 × years)

Calorie Requirements for Women *continued*

| Height | Age | To Maintain Weight Activity Level* | | | To Lose Weight | |
		Low	Medium	High	1 Lb/ Week	2 Lb/ Week
	50	1590	1740	1880	1240	740
	60	1540	1680	1820	1180	680
	70	1490	1620	1760	1120	620
	80	1440	1570	1700	1070	570
	90	1380	1510	1640	1010	510
	100	1330	1450	1570	950	450
5'11"	20	1770	1930	2090	1430	930
	30	1710	1870	2030	1370	870
	40	1660	1810	1970	1310	810
	50	1610	1760	1900	1260	760
	60	1560	1700	1840	1200	700
	70	1510	1650	1780	1150	650
	80	1460	1590	1720	1090	590
	90	1400	1530	1660	1030	530
	100	1350	1480	1600	980	480

*Low activity = 110% of basal energy expenditure (BEE); medium activity = 120% of basal energy expenditure (BEE); high activity = 130% of basal energy expenditure (BEE); BEE = $655 + (9.6 \times kg) + (1.7 \times cm) - (4.7 \times years)$

Calorie Requirements for Men

| Height | Age | To Maintain Weight Activity Level* | | | To Lose Weight | |
		Low	Medium	High	1 Lb/ Week	2 Lb/ Week
5'1"	20	1860	2030	2200	1530	1030
	30	1790	1950	2110	1450	950
	40	1710	1870	2030	1370	870
	50	1640	1790	1940	1290	790
	60	1560	1710	1850	1210	710
	70	1490	1630	1760	1130	630
	80	1420	1540	1670	1040	540
	90	1340	1460	1580	960	460
	100	1270	1380	1500	880	380
5'2"	20	1900	2070	2250	1570	1070
	30	1830	1990	2160	1490	990
	40	1750	1910	2070	1410	910
	50	1680	1830	1980	1330	830
	60	1600	1750	1890	1250	750
	70	1530	1670	1810	1170	670
	80	1450	1590	1720	1090	590
	90	1380	1500	1630	1000	500
	100	1300	1420	1540	920	420
5'3"	20	1930	2110	2280	1610	1110
	30	1860	2030	2200	1530	1030
	40	1780	1940	2110	1440	940
	50	1710	1860	2020	1360	860
	60	1630	1780	1930	1280	780
	70	1560	1700	1840	1200	700
	80	1480	1620	1750	1120	620
	90	1410	1540	1660	1040	540
	100	1330	1460	1580	960	460
5'4"	20	1970	2150	2330	1650	1150
	30	1890	2070	2240	1570	1070
	40	1820	1980	2150	1480	980

*Low activity = 110% of basal energy expenditure (BEE); medium activity = 120% of basal energy expenditure (BEE); high activity = 130% of basal energy expenditure (BEE); BEE = 66 + (13.7 × kg) + (5. × cm) − (6.8 × years)

Calorie Requirements for Men *continued*

Height	Age	To Maintain Weight Activity Level*			To Lose Weight	
		Low	Medium	High	1 Lb/ Week	2 Lb/ Week
	50	1740	1900	2060	1400	900
	60	1670	1820	1970	1320	820
	70	1590	1740	1880	1240	740
	80	1520	1660	1800	1160	660
	90	1450	1580	1710	1080	580
	100	1370	1490	1620	990	490
5'5"	20	2010	2190	2370	1690	1190
	30	1930	2120	2280	1620	1120
	40	1860	2030	2190	1530	1030
	50	1780	1940	2110	1440	940
	60	1710	1860	2020	1360	860
	70	1630	1780	1930	1280	780
	80	1560	1700	1840	1200	700
	90	1480	1620	1750	1120	620
	100	1410	1540	1660	1040	540
5'6"	20	2040	2230	2420	1730	1230
	30	1970	2150	2330	1650	1150
	40	1890	2070	2240	1570	1070
	50	1820	1990	2150	1490	990
	60	1750	1900	2060	1400	900
	70	1670	1820	1970	1320	820
	80	1600	1740	1890	1240	740
	90	1520	1660	1800	1160	660
	100	1450	1580	1710	1080	580
5'7"	20	2080	2270	2460	1770	1270
	30	2010	2190	2370	1690	1190
	40	1930	2110	2280	1610	1110
	50	1860	2030	2190	1530	1030
	60	1780	1940	2120	1440	940
	70	1710	1860	2020	1360	860

*Low activity = 110% of basal energy expenditure (BEE); medium activity = 120% of basal energy expenditure (BEE); high activity = 130% of basal energy expenditure (BEE); BEE = 66 + (13.7 × kg) + (5. × cm) − (6.8 × years)

Calorie Requirements for Men continued

| Height | Age | To Maintain Weight Activity Level* | | | To Lose Weight | |
		Low	Medium	High	1 Lb/ Week	2 Lb/ Week
	80	1630	1780	1930	1280	780
	90	1560	1700	1840	1200	700
	100	1480	1620	1750	1120	620
5'8"	20	2120	2310	2500	1810	1310
	30	2040	2230	2420	1730	1230
	40	1970	2150	2330	1650	1150
	50	1890	2070	2240	1570	1070
	60	1820	1980	2150	1480	980
	70	1740	1900	2060	1400	900
	80	1670	1820	1970	1320	820
	90	1600	1740	1890	1240	740
	100	1520	1660	1800	1160	660
5'9"	20	2160	2350	2550	1850	1350
	30	2080	2270	2460	1770	1270
	40	2010	2190	2370	1690	1190
	50	1930	2120	2280	1620	1120
	60	1860	2030	2190	1530	1030
	70	1780	1940	2110	1440	940
	80	1710	1860	2020	1360	860
	90	1630	1780	1930	1280	780
	100	1560	1700	1840	1200	700
5'10"	20	2190	2390	2590	1890	1390
	30	2120	2310	2500	1810	1310
	40	2040	2230	2410	1730	1230
	50	1970	2150	2330	1650	1150
	60	1890	2070	2240	1570	1070
	70	1820	1980	2150	1480	980
	80	1740	1900	2060	1400	900
	90	1670	1820	1970	1320	820
	100	1590	1740	1880	1240	740

*Low activity = 110% of basal energy expenditure (BEE); medium activity = 120% of basal energy expenditure (BEE); high activity = 130% of basal energy expenditure (BEE); BEE = 66 + (13.7 × kg) + (5. × cm) − (6.8 × years)

Calorie Requirements for Men *continued*

Height	Age	To Maintain Weight Activity Level*			To Lose Weight	
		Low	Medium	High	1 Lb/ Week	2 Lb/ Week
5'11"	20	2240	2440	2640	1940	1440
	30	2160	2360	2560	1860	1360
	40	2090	2280	2470	1780	1280
	50	2010	2200	2380	1700	1200
	60	1940	2110	2290	1610	1110
	70	1860	2030	2200	1530	1030
	80	1790	1950	2110	1450	950
	90	1710	1870	2020	1370	870
	100	1640	1790	1940	1290	790
6'0"	20	2270	2480	2690	1980	1480
	30	2200	2400	2600	1900	1400
	40	2130	2320	2510	1820	1320
	50	2050	2240	2420	1740	1240
	60	1980	2160	2330	1660	1160
	70	1900	2080	2250	1580	1080
	80	1830	1990	2160	1490	990
	90	1750	1910	2070	1410	910
	100	1680	1830	1980	1330	830
6'1"	20	2320	2530	2740	2030	1530
	30	2240	2450	2650	1950	1450
	40	2170	2370	2560	1870	1370
	50	2090	2280	2470	1780	1280
	60	2020	2200	2390	1700	1200
	70	1940	2120	2300	1620	1120
	80	1870	2040	2210	1540	1040
	90	1790	1960	2120	1460	960
	100	1720	1880	2030	1380	880
6'2"	20	2360	2580	2790	2080	1580
	30	2290	2500	2700	2000	1500
	40	2210	2410	2620	1910	1410

*Low activity = 110% of basal energy expenditure (BEE); medium activity = 120% of basal energy expenditure (BEE); high activity = 130% of basal energy expenditure (BEE); BEE = 66 + (13.7 × kg) + (5. × cm) − (6.8 × years)

Calorie Requirements for Men *continued*

| Height | Age | To Maintain Weight Activity Level* | | | To Lose Weight | |
		Low	Medium	High	1 Lb/ Week	2 Lb/ Week
	50	2140	2330	2530	1830	1330
	60	2060	2250	2440	1750	1250
	70	1990	2170	2350	1670	1170
	80	1910	2090	2260	1590	1090
	90	1840	2010	2170	1510	1010
	100	1760	1920	2080	1420	920
6'3"	20	2410	2630	2850	2130	1630
	30	2340	2550	2760	2050	1550
	40	2260	2470	2680	1970	1470
	50	2190	2390	2590	1890	1390
	60	2110	2310	2500	1810	1310
	70	2040	2230	2410	1730	1230
	80	1970	2140	2320	1640	1140
	90	1890	2060	2230	1560	1060
	100	1820	1980	2150	1480	980

*Low activity = 110% of basal energy expenditure (BEE); medium activity = 120% of basal energy expenditure (BEE); high activity = 130% of basal energy expenditure (BEE); BEE = 66 + (13.7 × kg) + (5. × cm) − (6.8 × years)

Consume at least 1,000 calories each day to satisfy your nutrient requirements. If calories are restricted below 1,000, the weight loss will be from muscle and fat. Your goal is to decrease body fat.

Frequently people will make the decision to lose weight through severe calorie restriction. It is important to distinguish between weight loss that is due to calorie restriction and weight loss that is due to water loss or diuresis. Seven patients were admitted to the General Clinical Research Center to consume diets containing an average of 600 calories. Their first-morning weight averaged 237 pounds. Sodium in their diet and urine was measured in order to determine how much weight change was due to calorie restriction and how much was due to water loss.

The average weight loss for the first day was three pounds. Two pounds were lost for each day on the second and third day. The patients lost one pound each day for the following four days. After the first week of severe dieting, the weight loss leveled off to two or three pounds per week, which simply reflected calorie restriction.

There was a large variation in individual weight loss. Those patients who normally consumed large amounts of salt lost up to fifteen pounds while those who consumed normal amounts of salt lost three pounds for the first week. If you lose more than six pounds during the first week of dieting, know that your sodium intake is much too high!

You can determine the grams of protein, carbohydrate, and fat equal to a specific number of calories by using the table on page 69. Well-balanced diets contain a calorie distribution of 15 percent protein, 55 percent carbohydrate, and 30 percent fat. An 1,800-calorie diet would contain 68 grams of protein, 248 grams of carbohydrate, and 60 grams of fat. Decreasing fat to 30 percent and increasing carbohydrate to 55 percent are major nutrition goals for most people.

If you have elevated blood fats and are overweight, you can significantly reduce your risk for heart disease by changing your calorie distribution to 15 percent protein, 65 percent carbohydrate, and 20 percent fat. An 1,800-calorie diet would contain 68 grams of protein, 293 grams of carbohydrate, and 40 grams of fat.

Grams of Protein, Carbohydrate, and Fat for Varied Calorie Distributions

Calories	Protein (15%), Grams	Carbohydrate (55%), Grams	Fat (30%), Grams
800	30	110	27
900	34	124	30
1000	38	138	33
1100	41	151	37
1200	45	165	40
1300	49	179	43
1400	53	193	47
1500	56	206	50
1600	60	220	53
1700	64	234	57
1800	68	248	60
1900	71	261	63
2000	75	275	67
2100	79	289	70
2200	83	303	73
2300	86	316	77
2400	90	330	80
2500	94	344	83
2600	98	358	87
2700	101	371	90
2800	105	385	93
2900	109	399	97
3000	113	413	100

Grams of Protein, Carbohydrate, and Fat for Varied Calorie Distributions

Calories	Protein (15%), Grams	Carbohydrate (65%), Grams	Fat (20%), Grams
800	30	130	18
900	34	146	20
1000	38	163	22
1100	41	179	24
1200	45	195	27
1300	49	211	29
1400	53	228	31
1500	56	244	33
1600	60	260	36
1700	64	276	38
1800	68	293	40
1900	71	309	42
2000	75	325	44
2100	79	341	47
2200	83	358	49
2300	86	374	51
2400	90	390	53
2500	94	406	56
2600	98	423	58
2700	101	439	60
2800	105	455	62
2900	109	471	64
3000	113	488	67

Calorie requirements can be met through numerous combinations of protein, carbohydrate, and fat. The total number of calories determines if you will lose, maintain, or gain weight. The numbers are much more meaningful when they can be related to food decisions. Consider the comparison of the following two 500-calorie meals.

	Meal A	Meal B
protein	15%	15%
carbohydrate	55%	65%
fat	30%	20%

Food	Portion	Portion
roast beef	2 oz	2 oz
mayonnaise	1 tsp	
mustard		1 tsp
whole-wheat bread	2 slices	2 slices
vegetable soup	8 oz	8 oz
banana	4 oz	4 oz
grapes		3 oz

Substituting mayonnaise, which is high in fat, with mustard reduces the fat content of the meal from 30 to 20 percent. Three ounces of grapes are added to Meal B to increase the carbohydrate from 55 percent to 65 percent.

Decreasing fat is the most efficient way to decrease calories. Protein and carbohydrate each contain four calories per gram while fat contains nine calories per gram. Fat contains more than twice the calories per gram of protein and carbohydrate. Count fat grams, as found in the food tables in the chapter on food composition, as an alternative to counting calories. Use the following table to determine the amount of fat per calorie level. If you require 1,650 calories, fat should not exceed 59 grams if the total diet has a calorie distribution of 30 percent fat.

Grams of Fat (30%) for Multiple Calorie Levels

Calories	00	10	20	30	40	50	60	70	80	90
800	27	28	29	30	31	32	33	35	36	37
900	30	31	32	33	34	36	37	38	39	40
1000	33	34	36	37	38	39	40	41	42	43
1100	37	38	39	40	41	42	43	45	46	47
1200	40	41	42	43	44	46	47	48	49	50
1300	43	44	46	47	48	49	50	51	52	53
1400	47	48	49	50	51	52	53	55	56	57
1500	50	51	52	53	54	56	57	58	59	60
1600	53	54	56	57	58	59	60	61	62	63
1700	57	58	59	60	61	62	63	65	66	67
1800	60	61	62	63	64	66	67	68	69	70
1900	63	64	66	67	68	69	70	71	72	73
2000	67	68	69	70	71	72	73	75	76	77
2100	70	71	72	73	74	76	77	78	79	80
2200	73	74	76	77	78	79	80	81	82	83
2300	77	78	79	80	81	82	83	85	86	87
2400	80	81	82	83	84	86	87	88	89	90
2500	83	84	86	87	88	89	90	91	92	93
2600	87	88	89	90	91	92	93	95	96	97
2700	90	91	92	93	94	96	97	98	99	100
2800	93	94	96	97	98	99	100	101	102	103
2900	97	98	99	100	101	102	103	105	106	107
3000	100	101	102	103	104	106	107	108	109	110

If you have elevated blood fats, try a diet with 20 percent of the calories coming from fat. Most people need to adjust calorie distribution by decreasing fat and increasing carbohydrate. It is difficult to accomplish a dietary distribution of 30 percent fat, let alone 20 percent. While many individual meals can be low in fat, many meals can be very high in fat.

Eating out a couple of times each week can greatly increase the fat in your diet. About 50 percent of the calories in fast-food meals are derived from fat. Over the next decade, the level of dietary fat may change by the introduction of fat substitutes. However, be realistic and accept personal responsibility for the change. Change is a gradual process.

Grams of Fat (20%) for Multiple Calorie Levels

Calories	00	10	20	30	40	50	60	70	80	90
800	18	18	18	18	19	19	19	19	20	20
900	20	20	20	21	21	21	21	22	22	22
1000	22	22	23	23	23	23	24	24	24	24
1100	24	25	25	25	25	26	26	26	26	26
1200	27	27	27	27	28	28	28	28	28	29
1300	29	29	29	30	30	30	30	30	31	31
1400	31	31	32	32	32	32	32	33	33	33
1500	33	34	34	34	34	34	35	35	35	35
1600	36	36	36	36	36	37	37	37	37	38
1700	38	38	38	38	39	39	39	39	40	40
1800	40	40	40	41	41	41	41	42	42	42
1900	42	42	43	43	43	43	44	44	44	44
2000	44	45	45	45	45	46	46	46	46	46
2100	47	47	47	47	48	48	48	48	48	49
2200	49	49	49	50	50	50	50	50	51	51
2300	51	51	52	52	52	52	52	53	53	53
2400	53	54	54	54	54	54	55	55	55	55
2500	56	56	56	56	56	57	57	57	57	58
2600	58	58	58	58	59	59	59	59	60	60
2700	60	60	60	61	61	61	61	62	62	62
2800	62	62	63	63	63	63	64	64	64	64
2900	64	65	65	65	65	66	66	66	66	66
3000	67	67	67	67	68	68	68	68	68	69

A 1,650-calorie diet would contain 37 grams of fat. For comparison, consider that one Big Mac contains 34 grams of fat.

At times the many different types of fat may seem confusing. There are saturated fats in red meats, omega-3 fatty acids in fish, cholesterol in egg yolks, and polyunsaturated fats in vegetable oils. The rule of thumb for selecting fat is to answer the question, "Can you pour it?" If the fat is liquid at room temperature, it is high in polyunsaturated fats and is better for you than butter, lard, and some margarines that are solid at room temperature. If the fat is solid, it is high in saturated fat. All fats are high in calories!

Cholesterol

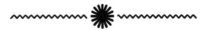

C holesterol is just one type of fat found in foods and the blood. An optimal fasting blood value is 160 to 200 milligrams per deciliter (mg/dl). A high blood cholesterol is strongly associated with increased risk for developing heart and blood vessel disease.

Egg yolks and liver are the major food sources for cholesterol. Vegetable oils are advertised as being special because they do not contain cholesterol. All vegetable oils do not contain cholesterol but they are still 100 percent fat!

Your body may be your major source of cholesterol because it can make the equivalent of two dozen eggs' worth of cholesterol from sugar each day. Fluctuations in blood sugar and blood fat can be reduced by distributing foods evenly throughout the day.

Consume small, frequent meals and snacks. In graduate school at the University of Kentucky, I did my thesis on the effects of different foods on fat synthesis in rats. To identify the food effects, fat synthesis was maximized by using a meal feeding pattern. The rats had access to food for three hours each morning. Regardless of the food source, fat synthesis was greatest when the rats were given one large meal each day. The practice of skipping meals and then eating one large meal greatly increases fat synthesis.

You are a dynamic living system. Your body is constantly changing. It is extremely important to make blood cholesterol, triglycerides, and glucose assessments after not eating for twelve hours. It is normal for blood sugars and fats to increase significantly after eating. The more you eat, the more the parameters will increase. Consuming small amounts of food will decrease the postprandial increase of blood sugars and fats.

If you have a high blood cholesterol and have a family history of heart disease, your doctor will probably perform additional blood tests. Your blood contains substances that transport different kinds of fat throughout the body. These are called lipoproteins.

It can be confusing to sort out the different types of lipoproteins. It is best to start with a familiar example. To make chicken soup you throw a chicken into a pot of water and boil it. You take out the bones and pour the soup into a big jar. As it cools, the soup separates into layers. The fat rises to the top. The fat is lighter or less dense than the broth and thus separates out.

Analyzing blood for lipoproteins is similar to making chicken soup. The lipoproteins separate out based on their density. The *h*igh-*d*ensity *l*ipoprotein (HDL) is the heaviest and settles to the bottom. The *l*ow-*d*ensity *l*ipoprotein (LDL) settles in the middle. The *v*ery-*l*ow-*d*ensity *l*ipoprotein (VLDL) is the lightest, so it rises to the top. Just like chicken soup, the good stuff (HDL) is on the bottom and the bad stuff (VLDL) is on the top.

The HDL prevents the accumulation of fat. Women and athletes tend to have higher levels of HDL. Smokers have low levels of HDL. The LDL carries cholesterol in the blood and is associated with the accumulation of fatty materials in artery walls. The VLDL carries another type of fat called triglycerides.

While a normal blood cholesterol is 160 to 200 mg/dl, over half of the American adult population has a blood cholesterol greater than 200 mg/dl. We have a long way to go to achieve optimal health in America.

Sodium and Potassium

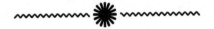

Many people who have high blood pressure are sensitive to salt (sodium chloride). Sodium and potassium are both minerals that influence blood pressure. Sodium tends to increase blood pressure while potassium tends to decrease blood pressure.

This is supported by epidemiological studies comparing reduced blood pressure in populations that consume small amounts of salt with Western populations that consume more salt. Western populations have a much higher incidence of high blood pressure.

The body is working to achieve a balance between dietary intake and the urinary excretion of salts. When sodium ingestion exceeds the kidneys' capability to excrete it, sodium will be retained by the body. This leads to water retention. Fluid expansion leads to the secretion of chemical substances that increase blood pressure.

Sodium balance can be normalized by decreasing intake or increasing output. Medications called diuretics are frequently used to increase the urinary excretion of sodium.

However, over time there may be significant side effects to taking diuretics. The mechanism for ridding the body of excess sodium also gets rid of potassium. It is common for a person taking diuretics to require additional potassium also. Some recently developed diuretics have potassium sparing qualities. Your doctor will check your blood potassium to determine if you require supplemental potassium.

Ordinary table salt, or sodium chloride (NaCl), is a major dietary source of sodium. One teaspoon of salt weighing 6 grams contains 2.3 grams of sodium and 3.7 grams of chloride. Your daily requirement of 0.5 grams of sodium is only a fraction of the average intake of 4 grams of sodium. Four grams of sodium equal 10 grams of table salt.

Fruits, vegetables, meats, and dairy products are significant sources of dietary potassium. People normally consume 2 grams of potassium each day. The average person consumes twice as much sodium as potassium. An optimal ratio for the general public would be one to one. If you have high blood pressure, it might be better to reduce the sodium potassium ratio further. In the chapter on food composition you will learn how to achieve this by adding the Heart Factor of foods.

Sometimes people use salt substitutes or potassium chloride (KCl). One teaspoon of potassium chloride weighing 6 grams contains 3.1 grams of potassium and 2.9 grams of chloride. Using salt substitutes can be very dangerous when used in combination with some medicines. As you will note, salt substitutes are labeled with the sound advice, "Consult a physician before using any salt substitute." Also, potassium chloride tastes very bitter and leaves an aftertaste. Potassium from food is the best alternative.

It is estimated that 39 percent of patients with hypertension could control blood pressure with a sodium intake below 1.1 grams per day and about one third who have mild hypertension could control their blood pressure with a sodium intake of 1.7 grams per day or less. It takes time and energy to learn to make low-sodium, high-potassium food choices. However, there are long-term benefits to becoming an expert!

Food Composition

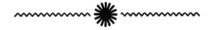

Food is a complex mixture of many nutrients. When selecting foods for health, you may try to add and determine total calories, milligrams of sodium and potassium, grams of protein, carbohydrate, fat, and fiber. This is fine and dandy if you are a nutritionist and enjoy making sense of all those numbers. In the real world, all that math is too confusing and time-consuming.

Rather than counting everything, set priorities. Focus on what is most important. Sodium tends to increase blood pressure, while potassium tends to decrease blood pressure. Therefore, it is important to know that you are consuming about 2 grams of potassium for every gram of sodium. It is simply a matter of consulting the food tables and adding the amounts corresponding to the foods you consume.

People normally consume about twenty to thirty foods each day. Keeping track of so many numbers is not much fun. It's time for a shortcut! Add the Heart Factor of foods. At times, sodium and potassium are expressed in milliequivalents (mEq) versus milligrams. The Heart Factor (HF) equals the mEq of sodium minus the mEq of potassium.

Heart Factor = (mg sodium/23.0) − (mg potassium/39.1)

A food that is high in sodium will have a positive Heart Factor, while a food that is high in potassium will have a negative Heart Factor. Select food combinations in which the high-sodium foods are balanced by an equal amount of potassium. The total Heart Factor should equal zero or less. Compare the following breakfast meals.

Food	Portion	HF
shredded wheat	1½ oz	−4
skim milk	8 oz	−4
banana	1 medium	+ −11
HEART FACTOR FOR MEAL		−19

Food	Portion	HF
English muffin	1 medium	2
peanut butter	1 oz	3
orange juice	6 oz	+ −5
HEART FACTOR FOR MEAL		0

Food	Portion	HF
biscuit	1 oz	7
sausage links	2 oz	38
grapefruit juice	6 oz	+ −9
HEART FACTOR FOR MEAL		36

Potassium-containing salt substitutes are no substitute for the nutritious qualities of potassium-containing foods. Fruits and vegetables, while high in potassium, are also low in fat, high in fiber, and high in essential vitamins. Dairy products, also high in potassium, are good sources of protein and calcium.

It is also important to count grams of fat. Your fat intake should range from 20 to 30 percent of your total calories. Consult the chapter on calories to estimate your calorie requirement. Consult pages 69 and 70 to determine an acceptable range of grams of fat to consume. For example, an 1,800-calorie diet should contain 40 to 60 grams of fat. Next, consult the food composition tables to determine the grams of fat in each food. Be sure to include the fat used in food preparation!

By counting the Heart Factor, you will find the math of keeping your sodium and potassium intake simplified. Counting the grams of fat can also be simplified. An asterisk (*) has been placed next to the Heart Factors of foods having 20 percent or more calories derived from fat. Count the grams of fat of only the foods having the asterisk. You will be on target if that sum equals the grams of fat equal to 20 percent of your calorie requirement.

Your fat intake will be more than 20 percent because you won't actually go through the mechanics of adding up the fat of the lower-fat foods. However, you will have set priorities by counting the grams of fat in the higher-fat foods. This method of calculating fat will be fast, easy, and accurate. You will be on target.

Studying the Heart Factor of foods is a quick way to compare many foods. Foods are first divided into the basic food groups. The food groups are subdivided into smaller food categories. Foods are listed alphabetically under each group.

I. FRUITS AND VEGETABLES

In this group are fruits, juices, soups, and vegetables. Fruits and vegetables are wonderful foods! They are low in fat, low in sodium, and high in potassium. In most cases the Heart Factor will be a negative number. They are packed with minerals, vitamins, and fiber essential for good health.

Fruits and vegetables are also high in vitamin C. If the food "keeps its color," it is high in vitamin C. Foods high in vitamin C are cantaloupe, grapefruit, oranges, strawberries, tangerines, broccoli, cabbage, tomatoes, and spinach. Apples, bananas, pineapple, and green beans, foods that turn brown when exposed to the air, contain less vitamin C.

Fresh fruits and vegetables are conveniently packaged. You can prepare the exact amount you plan to eat. Cooking vegetables in the microwave is ideal as it is fast and does not require adding fat. If you have leftover vegetables, make soup.

II. BREADS AND STARCHES

Breads and starches provide carbohydrate, minerals, B vitamins, fiber, and protein. Many people think that bread is "bad." Nothing smells or tastes as good as bread straight from the oven. Bread gets a bad name because it's something on which to put lots of margarine or butter. To reduce calories, try eating bread without the added fat. Apple butter, which does not contain any fat, can be an alternative choice.

Breads, cakes, cereals, chips and snacks, cookies, crackers, flour, rice, and pasta are in the bread food group. All breads and starches are a welcome choice for health. Sodium and fat vary significantly in this food group.

For example, consider the choices listed within the bread category. A slice of whole-wheat bread has a Heart Factor of 4 compared to a doughnut with a Heart Factor of 12. If you normally eat a doughnut, consider an English muffin, which has a Heart Factor of 2. The Heart Factor will help you to make food decisions.

III. MEATS

This food group includes beef, nuts, pork, poultry, and seafood. Foods from the meat group contain protein, potassium, and phosphorus. Trim meats of all fat. Do not use the chicken skin. Broil and bake meats. Don't fry any of these foods. Oils are liquid fat containing the same number of calories as lard or butter.

Cooking meats differently may be one of the most difficult habits to change. Be imaginative. Try adding fruits and spices. Fruits complement meats while keeping them moist. Spices improve flavor without adding calories or sodium. Cook chicken with orange slices and/or ginger, for example. Consult the chapter on recipes to discover alternatives to the salt shaker.

IV. DAIRY PRODUCTS

Skim milk, cottage cheese, yogurt, and cheese provide the body with needed calcium, vitamin D, and protein. Use low-fat dairy products. The fat in whole milk or cream provides extra calories. If skim milk is completely unacceptable, use a smaller portion of 2 percent fat milk. Don't exclude dairy products.

V. MISCELLANEOUS

Thinking of the thousands of foods available, we quickly realize that many are missing from the basic four groups. These foods are beverages, candy, condiments, fats, sugars, and seasonings.

Experiment with combinations to increase variety in your diet. Your ultimate goal is to normalize weight and include all foods in your diet.

To become familiar with the food composition table, consider the nutrient content of the "diet sheet."

		HF	Calories	Fat
BREAKFAST:				
shredded wheat	1½ oz	−4	170	1.0
skim milk	8 oz	−4	86	0.2
banana	4 oz	−11	112	0.2
LUNCH:				
lettuce	2 oz	−2	9	0.2
tomato	2 oz	−4	14	0.1
cucumber	2 oz	−2	7	0.1
cottage cheese	3.3 oz	8	104	4.2
FRUIT BREAK:				
orange	4 oz	−5	64	0.2
SUPPER:				
chicken	3.3 oz	−6	96	1.5
potato	4 oz	−12	91	0.1
broccoli	3.3 oz	−6	24	0.3
FRUIT BREAK:				
apple	4 oz	−3	70	0.4
	TOTAL	−51	847	8.5

Group I Fruits and Vegetables

Food	HF	G	Oz	Cal	Na	K	Fat	%Fat
FRUIT, CANNED:								
applesauce	−2	90	3	39	2	70	0.2	4
applesauce, sweet	−1	90	3	86	2	59	0.1	1
fruit salad, "lite"	−4	90	3	58	5	148	0.1	1
pineapple	−3	90	3	56	1	132	0.1	1
FRUIT, FRESH:								
apple	−3	120	4	70	1	132	0.4	5
apricot	−6	90	3	50	1	253	0.2	3
banana	−11	120	4	112	1	444	0.2	2
blackberries	−4	90	3	43	1	153	0.8	17
blueberries	−2	90	3	57	1	73	0.5	7
boysenberries	−4	90	3	38	1	138	0.3	6
cantaloupe	−7	120	4	40	14	276	0.1	3
cherries	−4	90	3	68	2	172	0.3	4
gooseberries	−4	90	3	32	1	140	0.2	5
grapefruit	−4	120	4	53	1	162	0.1	2
grapes	−4	90	3	68	3	142	0.9	12
honeydew melon	−7	120	4	41	14	301	0.4	8
kiwifruit	−7	90	3	57	5	298	0.4	6
orange	−5	120	4	64	1	204	0.2	3
peach	−6	120	4	40	14	276	0.1	3
pear	−4	120	4	74	2	155	0.5	6
plum	−4	90	3	45	2	150	0.1	2
raisins	−5	30	1	95	9	218	0.1	1
strawberries	−4	120	4	43	1	174	0.6	13
tangerine	−3	120	4	59	2	132	0.2	4
watermelon	−6	240	8	67	2	240	0.5	6
JUICE *(6-oz cup)*:								
apple	−5	180	6	86	2	182	0.0	0
apricot nectar	−7	180	6	108	0	272	0.2	2
cranberry	0	180	6	121	2	18	0.2	1
grape	−5	180	6	130	2	216	0.5	4
grapefruit	−9	180	6	74	4	356	0.2	2
orange	−9	180	6	83	2	360	0.4	4

Group I Fruits and Vegetables *continued*

Food	HF	G	Oz	Cal	Na	K	Fat	%Fat
pineapple	−6	180	6	101	2	252	0.2	2
prune	−11	180	6	142	4	423	0.2	1
V-8	13	180	6	40	536	395	0.1	2

SOUP *(1 cup):*

Food	HF	G	Oz	Cal	Na	K	Fat	%Fat
asparagus, milk	38*	240	8	142	1046	295	5.8	37
bean w. pork	32*	240	8	158	967	379	5.5	31
beef broth	30	240	8	31	782	130	0.0	0
beef noodle	38*	240	8	67	917	77	2.6	35
bouillon cube	52*	5	¼	6	1200	5	0.2	21
celery, milk	37*	240	8	166	1018	283	9.1	50
chicken broth	31	240	8	22	722	24	0.0	0
chicken gumbo	39*	240	8	55	950	108	1.4	23
chicken noodle	45*	240	8	74	1063	53	2.4	29
chicken w. rice	37*	240	8	46	917	98	1.2	24
pea soup	33	240	8	127	881	192	2.2	15
tomato, milk	34*	240	8	170	1013	401	6.7	35
tomato soup	35*	240	8	77	919	180	2.4	28
turkey noodle	41*	240	8	77	998	77	2.9	34
vegetable beef	41*	240	8	77	1025	156	2.2	25

VEGETABLES, CANNED:

Food	HF	G	Oz	Cal	Na	K	Fat	%Fat
asparagus	5	90	3	22	212	149	0.4	15
beets	5	90	3	33	212	150	0.1	2
carrots	7	90	3	25	212	108	0.2	6
corn	7	90	3	85	212	87	0.7	8
green beans	7	90	3	22	212	86	0.2	8
kidney beans	6	90	3	104	320	306	0.5	4
lima beans	4	90	3	80	212	200	0.2	2
peas	7	90	3	47	212	86	0.3	5
pork & beans	13*	90	3	106	417	189	2.3	20
spinach	7	90	3	19	288	234	0.4	17
water chestnuts	−7	60	2	113	4	272	0.9	7

*fat = 20 or more percent of calories

Group I Fruits and Vegetables *continued*

Food	HF	G	Oz	Cal	Na	K	Fat	%Fat
VEGETABLES, GREEN, FRESH OR FROZEN:								
artichokes	−8	90	3	41	39	387	0.2	4
asparagus	−4	90	3	20	1	165	0.2	8
avocadoes	−9*	60	2	105	2	362	9.8	84
broccoli	−6	90	3	24	9	240	0.3	10
cabbage	−5	90	3	23	18	210	0.2	7
celery	−2	60	2	11	58	175	0.1	5
collards	−1	90	3	33	0	47	0.6	17
cucumbers	−2	60	2	7	4	96	0.1	8
green beans	−3	90	3	23	4	136	0.2	7
lettuce	−2	60	2	9	7	84	0.2	12
lima beans	−10	90	3	96	1	380	0.5	4
peas	−5	90	3	59	1	176	0.4	5
spinach	−6	90	3	24	45	292	0.3	10
turnip greens	4	90	3	17	212	219	0.3	14
VEGETABLES, NOT GREEN, FRESH OR FROZEN:								
beets	−3	90	3	28	39	187	0.1	3
black-eyed peas	−6	90	3	114	35	303	0.4	3
carrots	−5	90	3	35	45	280	0.2	5
cauliflower	−9	90	3	26	14	360	0.2	6
corn	−4	90	3	85	0	149	0.9	10
mushrooms	−8	60	2	14	3	312	0.1	8
potatoes	−12	120	4	91	4	488	0.1	1
squash	−5	90	3	18	1	182	0.1	5
sweet potatoes	−7	120	4	136	12	292	0.5	3
tomatoes	−4	60	2	14	2	161	0.1	8
turnips	−4	90	3	26	44	241	0.2	6

Group II Breads and Starches

Food	HF	G	Oz	Cal	Na	K	Fat	%Fat
BREADS:								
bagel	8	55	1⅘	161	199	41	1.5	9
biscuit	7*	30	1	110	188	35	5.1	42
blueberry muffin	0*	60	2	167	69	132	5.6	30
cornbread	7*	40	1⅓	129	192	44	4.2	30
doughnut	12*	60	2	235	301	54	11.2	43
English muffin	2*	60	2	175	75	60	6.1	31
French bread	6	25	⅘	71	145	23	0.8	10
hamburger bun	10	40	1⅓	113	241	37	2.1	17
hot dog bun	9	40	1⅓	111	216	35	2.0	16
Italian bread	6	25	⅘	67	146	19	0.2	3
pancakes	18*	120	4	272	510	148	8.4	28
rye bread	5	25	⅘	63	139	36	0.3	4
waffles	20*	120	4	330	570	174	11.8	32
white bread	5	25	⅘	66	127	26	0.8	11
whole-wheat bread	4	25	⅘	63	132	68	0.8	11
CAKES:								
angel food	6	60	2	163	170	53	0.1	1
brownies	4*	60	2	305	151	114	18.8	55
chocolate, iced	4*	60	2	233	141	92	9.8	38
fruit cake	2*	60	2	239	116	140	9.9	37
gingerbread	1*	60	2	191	142	272	6.4	30
pound cake	4*	60	2	247	107	47	11.2	41
sponge, plain	3	60	2	179	100	52	3.4	17
yellow, plain	6*	60	2	219	155	47	7.6	31
CEREALS:								
All-Bran	8	45	1½	154	514	563	0.8	4
Bran Chex	9	45	1½	167	423	366	1.3	7
bran flakes	11	45	1½	164	416	289	0.8	4
Cheerios	17	45	1½	177	493	162	2.9	15
cornflakes	18	45	1½	168	452	54	0.2	1
Grapenuts	10	45	1½	169	317	153	0.2	1

*fat = 20 or more percent of calories

Group II Breads and Starches *continued*

Food	HF	G	Oz	Cal	Na	K	Fat	%Fat
grits, cooked†	−1	120	4	59	13	72	0.1	2
Nutri-Grain, Wheat	10	45	1½	172	310	124	0.5	3
oatmeal, cooked†	−2	120	4	66	2	73	1.2	16
Product 19	21	45	1½	172	522	71	0.3	2
raisin bran	8	45	1½	158	327	234	0.9	5
shredded wheat	−4	45	1½	170	5	164	1.0	5
Special K	17	45	1½	174	426	79	0.2	1
wheat germ	−9*	45	1½	171	1	351	4.9	26
CHIPS, SNACKS *(1 oz):*								
Cheese Puffs	16*	30	1	169	394	44	10.7	57
corn chips	8*	30	1	168	196	41	10.4	56
popcorn	−2	30	1	118	1	60	1.5	11
potato chips	4*	30	1	172	300	339	11.9	63
pretzels	21	30	1	115	504	39	1.4	11
COOKIES *(1 oz):*								
animal crackers	5*	30	1	130	121	28	3.1	22
chocolate chip	4*	30	1	159	104	35	9.0	51
coconut bars	0*	30	1	150	45	68	7.4	44
fig bars	2	30	1	114	96	88	2.1	17
gingersnaps	4	30	1	126	171	139	2.7	19
macaroons	−3*	30	1	146	11	139	6.9	42
molasses	4*	30	1	140	116	42	5.8	37
oatmeal	4*	30	1	137	115	33	5.3	35
peanut butter	6*	30	1	150	171	57	7.8	47
sandwich	6*	30	1	150	146	11	6.6	40
shortbread	5*	30	1	158	135	19	8.6	49
sugar wafers	2*	30	1	145	57	19	5.7	36
vanilla wafers	3*	30	1	139	76	22	4.8	31
CRACKERS *(1 oz):*								
cheese	14*	30	1	162	360	56	9.8	54
graham	5*	30	1	129	141	49	3.2	23

*fat = 20 or more percent of calories
†If salt is used in the preparation, the HF will equal 10.

Group II Breads and Starches *continued*

Food	HF	G	Oz	Cal	Na	K	Fat	%Fat
graham w. choc.	3*	30	1	152	122	97	7.2	42
Melba toast	0	30	1	113	23	68	1.5	12
oyster	16*	30	1	129	381	36	3.5	25
rice wafers	1	30	1	90	24	9	0.0	0
Ritz	12*	30	1	165	291	24	8.7	47
rye wafers	7	30	1	108	265	180	0.4	3
saltines	15*	30	1	128	360	36	3.6	25
soda, unsalted	9*	30	1	129	223	38	3.4	24
Waverly wafers	15*	30	1	135	360	26	6.0	40
wheat snacks	7*	30	1	140	196	53	5.9	38
FLOUR *(1 cup):*								
all-purpose	−3	112	4	400	3	106	1.1	2
cake	−2	100	3½	364	3	95	0.8	2
rye	−6	112	4	392	1	227	1.9	4
self-rising	50	112	4	436	1208	101	1.2	2
whole wheat	−11	120	4	400	4	444	1.4	3
PASTA, RICE, SPAGHETTI; COOKED *(½ cup):*								
macaroni & cheese	21*	100	3½	215	543	120	11.1	46
rice, brown†	−2	100	3½	106	3	64	0.6	5
rice, white†	−1	100	3½	124	2	28	0.6	5
spaghetti†	−1	100	3½	108	1	59	0.4	3
PIES:								
apple	5*	100	3½	243	153	85	10.1	37
Boston cream	4	60	2	161	112	53	3.2	18
chocolate cream	8*	100	3½	272	273	142	15.2	50
coconut	4*	100	3½	235	183	163	12.5	48
lemon meringue	7*	100	3½	254	186	44	9.4	33
pecan	7*	100	3½	430	221	123	22.9	48
pumpkin	5*	100	3½	213	214	160	11.2	47

*fat = 20 or more percent of calories
†If salt is used in the preparation, the HF will equal 10.

Group III Meats

Food	HF	G	Oz	Cal	Na	K	Fat	%Fat
BEEF *(average portion):*								
chuck, lean, raw	−7*	100	3½	155	60	370	7.4	43
chuck, lean, cooked	−4*	70	2½	144	46	249	6.7	42
corned beef	50*	70	2½	253	1218	105	21.3	76
hamburger, raw	−6*	100	3½	152	65	355	7.4	44
liver, cooked	−2*	100	3½	222	184	380	10.6	43
liver, raw	−1*	100	3½	135	136	281	3.8	25
spareribs, no fat	−6*	100	3½	187	65	355	11.6	56
NUTS *(1 oz):*								
almonds, plain	−6*	30	1	189	1	232	16.3	77
almonds, roasted	−3*	30	1	198	59	232	17.3	79
cashews	−7*	30	1	178	5	139	13.7	69
peanut butter	3*	30	1	185	182	201	14.8	72
peanuts, raw	−2*	30	1	181	0	61	14.5	72
peanuts, salted	0*	30	1	185	125	202	14.9	73
pecans	−5*	30	1	218	0	181	21.4	88
walnuts	−4*	30	1	210	0	136	19.4	83
PORK *(average portion):*								
bacon, cooked	6*	15	½	90	153	35	7.8	78
cold cuts	10*	30	1	123	255	45	11.5	84
ham, 5% fat	16*	30	1	39	434	106	1.5	35
ham, 11% fat	15*	30	1	55	400	101	3.2	53
pork, lean	−4*	100	3½	166	70	285	10.5	57
sausage, link	38*	68	2½	265	1020	228	21.6	73
POULTRY; NO SKIN *(average portion):*								
chicken, dark	−2*	100	3½	197	93	240	9.7	44
chicken, light	−6	100	3½	96	50	320	1.5	14
duck	−4*	100	3½	159	74	285	8.2	46
egg, one	1*	50	2	80	61	65	5.8	65
egg white, one	1	30	1	14	44	42	0.0	0
egg yolk, one	0*	20	1	72	10	20	6.0	75

*fat = 20 or more percent of calories

Group III Meats *continued*

Food	HF	G	Oz	Cal	Na	K	Fat	%Fat
turkey, dark	−4*	100	3½	179	79	290	7.2	36
turkey, light	−5	100	3½	148	64	305	3.2	19
SEAFOOD *(average portion):*								
carp	−5*	100	3½	140	51	285	7.1	46
clams	−1	100	3½	66	121	235	1.3	18
cod	−5	100	3½	73	86	339	0.3	4
crab, cooked	2*	100	3½	97	100	110	2.5	23
flounder	−6	100	3½	74	68	332	0.8	10
haddock	−3	100	3½	74	99	301	0.1	1
lobster	6*	100	3½	87	300	260	1.9	20
oysters	0	100	3½	66	73	110	1.2	16
perch	−3	100	3½	81	67	238	0.8	9
salmon	−8*	100	3½	202	48	391	13.6	61
scallops	−4	100	3½	76	150	420	0.2	2
shrimp	−1*	100	3½	95	140	258	2.2	21
smoked herring	24*	100	3½	205	720	285	12.9	57
tuna, oil packed	15*	100	3½	210	480	240	12.0	51
tuna, salt free	−5	100	3½	119	41	279	0.8	6
tuna, water packed	10	100	3½	111	405	284	0.9	7

*fat = 20 or more percent of calories

Group IV Dairy Products

Food	HF	G	Oz	Cal	Na	K	Fat	%Fat
CHEESE, NATURAL *(1 oz):*								
blue	16*	30	1	107	424	78	8.8	74
brick	6*	30	1	113	170	41	9.0	72
cheddar	9*	30	1	119	210	25	9.7	73
cottage	15	100	3½	90	406	96	1.9	19
cream	3*	30	1	114	75	22	11.3	89
feta	14*	30	1	80	339	19	6.4	72
Gouda	10*	30	1	108	249	36	8.4	70
mozzarella	4*	30	1	86	114	20	6.5	68
Parmesan	20*	30	1	119	486	28	7.8	59
Swiss	3*	30	1	115	79	33	8.4	65
CHEESE, PROCESSED *(1 oz):*								
American	18*	30	1	114	435	49	9.5	82
Swiss	16*	30	1	102	417	66	7.6	67
FROZEN DESSERTS:								
ice cream	−1*	60	2	127	24	67	7.5	53
ice milk, vanilla	−1*	60	2	86	48	121	2.6	27
MILK:								
buttermilk	5	240	8	86	312	336	0.2	3
evaporated	−1	30	1	23	35	99	0.1	4
half & half	0*	15	½	19	6	19	1.7	81
2% fat	−4*	240	8	120	120	371	4.6	35
chocolate, 1% fat	−4	240	8	153	146	409	2.4	14
skim	−4	240	8	86	125	348	0.2	3
skim, dry	−7	30	1	108	161	538	0.2	2
whole	−4*	240	8	187	120	346	11.8	57
YOGURT:								
fruit	−5	240	8	240	128	425	2.7	10
plain	−7*	240	8	151	168	561	3.7	22

*fat = 20 or more percent of calories

Group V Miscellaneous

Food	HF	G	Oz	Cals	Na	K	Fat	%Fat
BEVERAGES:								
beer†	−1	360	12	151	25	90	0.0	0
beer, "lite"†	−1	360	12	100	25	90	0.0	0
soda, sweet†	0	360	12	146	4	4	0.0	0
soda, diet	0	360	12	4	4	4	0.0	0
wine, table†	−2	120	4	120	5	96	0.0	0
CANDY (1 oz)‡:								
butterscotch	1	30	1	123	20	1	1.0	7
caramel	2*	30	1	124	64	58	3.0	22
chocolate disks	−1*	30	1	146	22	75	5.9	36
fudge	1*	30	1	126	57	44	3.7	26
jelly beans	0	30	1	113	3	0	0.2	1
marshmallows	0	30	1	100	12	2	0.0	0
milk chocolate	−2*	30	1	164	28	115	9.7	53
peanut bar	−3*	30	1	163	3	134	9.7	53
peanut brittle	−1*	30		133	9	45	3.1	21
CONDIMENTS, NOT SWEET (1 tbsp):								
mustard, yellow	8	15	½	13	188	20	0.0	0
olives, black (2)	7*	20	⅗	37	150	5	4.0	97
olives, green (3)	14*	13	⅖	15	312	7	1.6	96
pickle, dill (1)	57	100	3⅓	11	1428	200	0.2	16
pickle, kosher (1)	24	55	1⅘	7	581	51	0.1	13
soy sauce	43	18	½	12	1029	64	0.0	0
steak sauce	7	15	½	10	157	10	0.0	0
Tabasco sauce	1	5	¼	1	22	3	0.0	0
teriyaki sauce	29	18	½	16	690	41	0.0	0
tomato catsup	5	15	½	17	156	54	0.0	0
vinegar	0	15	½	4	0	15	0.0	0
Worcestershire sauce	3	15	½	12	147	120	0.0	0
CONDIMENTS, SWEET (1 tbsp)‡:								
apple butter	−1	15	½	29	0	38	0.1	4
honey	0	15	½	46	1	8	0.0	0

*fat = 20 or more percent of calories
†These beverages are low in sodium, low in fat, but high in sugar and extra calories. Limit intake
‡Candy and sweet condiments are low in sodium but high in sugar and extra calories. Limit intake.

Group V Miscellaneous *continued*

Food	HF	G	Oz	Cals	Na	K	Fat	%Fat
jam, low calorie	0	15	½	22	0	10	0.0	0
marmalade, orange	0	15	½	42	3	7	0.1	2
molasses	−7	15	½	36	6	225	0.0	0
preserves	0	15	½	41	2	9	0.0	0
sugar, brown	−1	15	½	58	3	35	0.0	0
sugar, white	0	30	1	119	0	0	0.0	0
FATS *(1 tbsp)*:								
blue cheese dress.	9*	15	½	80	201	4	8.5	96
butter	0*	15	½	110	2	3	12.2	99
corn oil	0*	15	½	134	2	3	14.9	100
margarine, salted	6*	15	½	110	148	3	12.2	99
mayonnaise	4*	15	½	109	105	8	11.8	98
olive oil	0*	15	½	135	0	0	14.0	100
safflower oil	0*	15	½	135	2	3	15.0	100
sour cream	0*	15	½	32	8	21	3.1	87
SALT *(1 tsp)*	100	6	0.2	0	2300	0	0.0	0
SEASONINGS, FRENCH's *(1 tsp)*:								
celery salt	65	5	0.2	0	1505	0	0.0	0
garlic salt	89	6	0.2	4	2050	0	0.0	0
lemon pepper	35	4	0.1	4	805	0	0.0	0
onion salt	69	5	0.2	4	1590	0	0.0	0
salad seasoning	27	4	0.1	4	630	0	0.0	0
seafood seasoning	61	5	0.2	0	1410	0	0.0	0
seasoning salt	56	4	0.1	2	1280	0	0.0	0
SEASONINGS, LAWRY's *(1 tsp)*:								
salad sprinkle	18	5	0.2	19	479	39	0.0	0
seasoning salt	48	4	0.1	2	1164	111	0.0	0
SEASONINGS, MCCORMICK's *(1 tsp)*:								
chili pepper	−1	2	0.1	8	0	44	0.0	0
lemon pepper	3	4	0.1	9	77	23	0.0	0
salt & spice	62	5	0.2	5	1435	23	0.0	0
Season-All	42	4	0.1	4	980	17	0.0	0

*fat = 20 or more percent of calories

The following seasonings can be used freely. Consult the chapter on recipes to find food and spice combinations.

allspice	celery seeds
cinnamon	chili powder
cloves	curry powder
ginger	garlic powder
nutmeg	mustard
pumpkin pie spice	onion powder
	oregano
	paprika
	pepper, black or cayenne
	poultry seasoning
	sage

Fiber

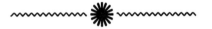

D ietary fiber is a complex mixture of plant substances
that man does not have the enzymes to digest. Cellu-
lose, hemicellulose, and lignins are common dietary fibers
that form the supportive cell walls of plants. In addition,
there are water-soluble dietary fibers such as gums and pec-
tins found in the endosperm of the plant seed.

People consuming diets high in water-soluble fibers may
decrease their blood cholesterol, blood triglycerides, and
blood sugars. If this is true, the risk for heart and blood
vessel disease would be correspondingly reduced. Experi-
ments to test the hypothesis are difficult to interpret because
the high-fiber diets are also very low in fats. The changes
observed may be more dependent on a low-fat diet than on
specific lipid-lowering attributes of fiber.

There are additional benefits to consuming a high-fiber
diet. Diets high in water-insoluble fibers adsorb water,
which increases stool bulk. This may contribute to an increased feeling of satiety. High-fiber diets are also beneficial
in the treatment of diverticulosis and constipation. The inci-

dence of some types of colon cancer may also be reduced when high-fiber diets are consumed.

Daily intakes for total dietary fiber are estimated at 10 grams for children, 12 grams for women, and 18 grams for men. The United States Department of Health and Human Services has recommended a daily intake of 30 grams of fiber. There is plenty of room for most people to increase their dietary-fiber intake by eating more vegetables, fruits, and whole-grain products. These foods have the added benefit in that they are also low in sodium, high in potassium, and low in fat.

Use the following table to estimate your normal dietary-fiber intake. Meats, dairy products, and fats are not listed because they do not contain any dietary fiber. Values are derived from food tables published by Dr. James W. Anderson in *Diabetes Care,* Vol. 1, No. 5, pages 293–302, 1978.

Fiber Content of Common Portions of Foods

		Plant Fiber		
Food	Grams	Total Grams	Soluble Grams	Insoluble Grams
BREADS & CRACKERS:				
graham crackers	30	3.0	0.1	2.9
rye bread	25	2.7	0.1	2.6
rye wafer	30	3.5	0.1	3.4
saltines	30	1.2	0.0	1.2
white bread	25	0.7	0.0	0.7
whole-wheat bread	25	2.4	0.1	2.3
CEREAL, FLOUR & GRAINS:				
All-Bran	45	14.9	0.4	14.5
cornflakes	45	5.0	1.5	3.5
flour, rye	100	13.9	0.4	13.5
flour, white	100	3.2	0.1	3.1
flour, whole wheat	100	9.5	0.3	9.2
grits, dry	30	3.2	1.0	2.2
oats, dry	30	2.7	0.9	1.8
rice, brown, dry	30	1.7	0.0	1.7
rice, white, dry	30	0.6	0.0	0.6
shredded wheat	45	5.5	0.2	5.3
spaghetti, dry	30	1.1	0.0	1.1
FRUITS:				
apple	120	4.1	2.4	1.7
apricot	90	1.5	0.9	0.6
banana	120	2.2	1.1	1.1
blackberries	90	4.5	0.8	3.7
cherries	90	1.1	0.4	0.7
grapefruit	120	1.6	1.1	0.5
grapes	90	0.7	0.2	0.5
melon	120	1.4	0.4	1.0
orange	120	2.5	1.9	0.6
peach	120	1.6	0.8	0.8
pear	120	2.9	0.7	2.2
pineapple	90	0.9	0.3	0.6

Fiber Content of Common Portions of Foods *continued*

Food	Grams	Plant Fiber		
		Total Grams	*Soluble* Grams	*Insoluble* Grams
plum	90	1.6	0.9	0.7
strawberries	120	2.5	1.0	1.5
tangerine	120	2.5	1.9	0.6
VEGETABLES, GREEN:				
asparagus	90	1.5	0.5	1.0
broccoli	90	3.7	2.3	1.4
cabbage	90	2.5	1.5	1.0
celery	60	1.8	0.5	1.3
cucumbers	60	0.9	0.5	0.4
green beans	90	3.1	1.1	2.0
greens	90	3.3	1.4	1.9
lettuce	60	0.9	0.4	0.5
lima beans	90	3.3	1.4	1.9
peas	90	7.0	2.7	4.3
VEGETABLES, NOT GREEN:				
beets	90	2.3	0.9	1.4
carrots	90	3.3	2.3	1.0
cauliflower	90	1.6	0.5	1.1
corn	90	4.2	1.3	2.9
kidney beans	90	4.3	0.5	3.8
popcorn	30	4.7	1.4	3.3
potatoes	120	4.2	2.4	1.8
squash	90	2.7	1.3	1.4
sweet potatoes	120	4.8	2.6	2.2
tomatoes	60	0.8	0.2	0.6
turnips	90	2.0	0.9	1.1
white beans	90	4.2	0.5	3.7

Vitamins and Minerals

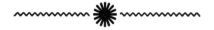

V itamins and minerals are nutrients needed in small amounts. The energy-providing nutrients of protein, carbohydrate, and fat are needed in much larger amounts. An 1,800-calorie diet may contain 68 grams of protein, 248 grams of carbohydrate, and 60 grams of fat. By comparison, vitamin and mineral requirements are usually in milligram (mg) or microgram (μg) amounts. There are 1,000 milligrams in a gram and 1,000 micrograms in a milligram.

According to the Surgeon General's Report on Nutrition and Health (1988), most Americans do not require vitamin and mineral supplements. An estimated 40 percent of Americans consume supplemental vitamins, minerals, or other dietary components at a cost of $2.7 billion per year. Toxicity has been reported for most minerals and trace elements, as well as some vitamins, indicating that excessive supplementation with these substances can be hazardous.

Food is the best way to get most nutrients. However, if you choose to use supplements, please do not exceed the recommended amounts. While it is reassuring to think that our food intake is adequate, there are times when supplementation of specific nutrients is appropriate.

Frequent blood donors, women of reproductive age, very young children, and strict vegetarians may require an iron supplement. In addition, people in these high-risk groups may require supplemental vitamin B_{12} and folic acid to prevent nutrient deficiency anemias.

Many people do not consume dairy products and may therefore need supplemental calcium to maintain the integrity of the skeletal system. Tums work very well as an economical and effective calcium supplement.

People who decrease their food intake for the purpose of weight reduction may require a daily mineral and vitamin supplement. Supplements should not exceed the recommended amounts.

Vitamins are organic substances. Vitamins are similar to the energy-providing nutrients in that they also contain carbon. Vitamins are classified as being water soluble or fat soluble. Water-soluble vitamins are excreted in the urine, while fat-soluble vitamins are stored in fatty tissues and the liver. The fat-soluble vitamins A, D, E, and K are stored in the liver and can be toxic if consumed in excessive amounts. The role of vitamins is to facilitate many chemical reactions in the body.

Minerals are inorganic substances. Trace minerals are a subgroup of minerals that are required in very small amounts. The role of minerals is similar to that of vitamins in that they facilitate many chemical reactions in the body.

The following table provides an overview of basic information about vitamins and minerals. Names and alternate names are given. It would be easier if only one name was used for each of the nutrients. Well, it just didn't work out that way. When reading food labels, you may find both names are used. The recommended daily dietary allowance for adults age 25–50 is listed next. These numbers come from the Committee on Dietary Allowances, Food and Nutrition Board, National Research Council: Recommended Dietary Allowances, ed. 10, Washington, D.C., 1989, National Academy of Sciences. The nutrient levels are designed for the maintenance of good nutrition of practically all healthy people in the United States. The recommendations are routinely evaluated and updated as scientific information is gathered.

The Committee on Dietary Allowances has also established estimated safe and adequate daily dietary intakes for selected vitamins and minerals. Estimated minimum requirements have been established for sodium, chloride, and potassium.

The major food source and function in the body for each vitamin and mineral are also listed. Food is a complex mixture of many nutrients. Variety in food selection is one of the best ways to guarantee that you are consuming adequate amounts of them. Vitamins and minerals are essential for the health of all cells.

To help you understand some of the information in the tables, try answering the following questions. The answers are found in the tables.

Match the Names:

Vitamin A	Ascorbic Acid
Vitamin B_1	Tocopherol
Vitamin B_6	Calciferol
Vitamin B_{12}	Retinol
Vitamin C	Thiamin
Vitamin D	Cobalamin
Vitamin E	Pyridoxine

Match the Mineral Name with the Chemical Symbol:

Calcium	Cu
Phosphorus	Se
Sodium	Mg
Potassium	P
Selenium	Ca
Iron	Na
Copper	K
Magnesium	Fe

True or false: The following vitamins are water soluble and excreted in the urine.

_____ Ascorbic Acid	_____ Pantothenic Acid
_____ Biotin	_____ Phylloquinone
_____ Calciferol	_____ Pyridoxine
_____ Choline	_____ Retinol
_____ Cobalamin	_____ Riboflavin
_____ Folic Acid	_____ Thiamine
_____ Niacin	_____ Tocopherol

Match the Nutrient with the Recommended Daily Allowance:

Calcium	5 mg
Iron	0.8–1.0 mg
Niacin	10–15 mg
Vitamin A	15–19 mg
Vitamin C	60 mg
Vitamin D	800–1200 mg

Recommended Daily Dietary Allowances—Revised 1989*

Designed for the maintenance of good nutrition of practically all healthy people in the United States

---

Fat-Soluble Vitamins

Vitamin A   retinol   800–1000 μg
  Source: liver, carrots, spinach, dairy products
  Function: normal growth, night vision, healthy tissue

Vitamin D   calciferol   5 μg
  Source: dairy products, cod liver oil, sunshine
  Function: growth and mineralization of bones

Vitamin E   tocopherol   8–10 mg
  Source: vegetable oils, green leafy vegetables
  Function: antioxidant for essential fatty acids

---

*Listed requirements are from the Committee on Dietary Allowances, Food and Nutrition Board, National Research Council: Recommended Dietary Allowances, ed. 10, Washington, D.C., 1989. National Academy of Sciences

Vitamin K   phylloquinone   65–80 μg
Source: green leafy vegetables, cereals
Function: blood clotting

Water-Soluble Vitamins

Vitamin C   ascorbic acid   60 mg
Source: citrus fruits, tomato, broccoli, cantaloupe, potatoes,
          strawberries
Function: healthy connective tissue, healthy skin

Vitamin B$_1$ thiamine   1.1–1.5 mg
Source: pork, liver, legumes, whole grains
Function: coenzyme, energy metabolism

Vitamin B$_2$ riboflavin   1.3–1.7 mg
Source: liver, dairy products, made by intestinal flora
Function: coenzyme, energy metabolism

Niacin   15–19 mg
Source: liver, peanuts, lean meat, grains, legumes
Function: coenzyme, energy metabolism

Vitamin B$_6$ pyridoxine   1.6–2.0 mg
Source: meats, vegetables, whole grain cereals
Function: coenzyme, energy metabolism

Folic Acid   folate, folacin   180–200 μg
Source: green vegetables, legumes, whole grain products
Function: cell division, growth

Vitamin B$_{12}$ cobalamin   2.0 μg
Source: meats, eggs, dairy products
Function: protein metabolism

Minerals

Calcium   Ca   800 mg
Source: dairy products, green leafy vegetables
Function: bone and teeth formation

Phosphorus   P   800 mg
Source: milk, cheese, meats, eggs
Function: bone and teeth formation, acid-base balance

Magnesium   Mg   280–350 mg
   Source: whole grains, green leafy vegetables, meats
   Function: protein synthesis, calcium balance

Iron   Fe   10–15 mg
   Source: liver, enriched grains, cooking in iron pot, prunes, green
        leafy vegetables
   Function: red blood cells

Zinc   Zn   12–15 mg
   Source: oysters, seafood, meats
   Function: insulin, wound healing

Trace Minerals

Iodine   I   150 µg
   Source: seafood, iodized salt, vegetables depending on soil
   Function: thyroid hormone

Selenium   Se   55–70 µg
   Source: seafood, liver
   Function: antioxidant balance of cells

Estimated Safe and Adequate Daily Dietary Intakes— Revised 1989*

Water-Soluble Vitamins

Biotin   30–100 µ g
   Source: legumes, vegetables, meats
   Function: protein metabolism, lipid synthesis

Pantothenic Acid   4–7 mg
   Source: widely distributed
   Function: energy metabolism, Coenzyme A

*Listed requirements are from the Committee on Dietary Allowances, Food and Nutrition Board, National Research Council: Recommended Dietary Allowances, ed. 10, Washington, D.C., 1989. National Academy of Sciences

---

Trace Minerals

Copper   Cu   1.5–3.0 mg
  Source: protein-containing foods
  Function: enzymes in oxygen transport

Manganese   Mn   2–5 mg
  Source: green leafy vegetables, nuts, grains
  Function: synthesis of lipids, energy metabolism

Fluoride   Fl   1.5–4.0 mg
  Source: fluoridated water
  Function: bone formation

Chromium   Cr   50–200 μg
  Source: meat, dairy products, whole grains
  Function: carbohydrate and lipid metabolism

Molybdenum   Mo   75–250 μg
  Source: dairy products, legumes, grains, organ meats
  Function: enzyme cofactor

Estimated Minimum Requirements—Revised 1989*

Minerals

Sodium   Na   500 mg (22 mEq)
  Source: common salt, garlic and onion salt, baking soda and pow-
          der, seasoned meats
  Function: acid-base balance, water balance

Chloride   Cl   750 mg
  Source: common salt, salt substitutes
  Function: acid-base, water balance

Potassium   K   2000 mg (51 mEq)
  Source: fruits, vegetables, milk, meats, salt substitutes
  Function: acid-base balance, water balance

*Listed requirements are from the Committee on Dietary Allowances, Food and Nutrition Board, National Research Council: Recommended Dietary Allowances, ed. 10, Washington, D.C., 1989. National Academy of Sciences

Food Decisions:
What? When? How Much?

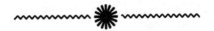

People have lost and gained back tons. Part of the reason for poor long-term success is the failure to recognize that food decisions are complex. Being "on" or "off" a diet leads to the belief that there is only one food decision to be made. It's not that simple. Through education you will have the information and confidence to make one hundred daily food decisions.

The first daily decision is to select the twenty to thirty foods and beverages you will consume. The second decision relates to food preparation. The third decision relates to food portions. Clearly if there are one hundred food decisions each day, this means three thousand decisions are made each month. This does not even consider the food decisions we make to not consume specific foods that are easily available. By now, you may be disheartened, thinking that it's all too much work. Be encouraged that the goal of achieving normal weight is accomplished through the sum of making many smaller decisions. A single food decision has little impact on achieving your ultimate health goal. Deciding to habitually and passively consume high-calorie foods will lead to failure.

Choosing among new and different things to eat is often an interesting journey through the many cultures of the world. Also, familiar foods in new combinations can be one way to select foods that you enjoy. I hesitate simply to distribute the magical "diet sheet" because it doesn't provide a sufficient opportunity for you to participate actively in food decisions. I respect individual choice. If you reduce the sugars and fats in your diet you can successfully achieve and maintain the right weight for optimal health. Increase variety as you successfully reach many of the small goals. This will help decrease boredom and promote your active participation.

Using a "small," "medium," and "large" portion size is arbitrary. To understand portion size, I asked twenty-four people to select a "medium" potato from a box of twenty-eight potatoes. The potatoes weighed six to eleven ounces each. The selected "medium" potatoes weighed six to ten ounces! So, the portion size was extremely individual. It was of interest to note that the size of the person was also directly related to the size of the selected potato. This also applied when people selected a "medium" apple, banana, or orange. It might be helpful to have a thin person select your portion!

The next food decision is food preparation. There are four calories per gram of protein and carbohydrate, seven calories per gram of alcohol, and nine calories per gram of fat. Calories can be effectively decreased by reducing fat. Fried chicken has twice the calories as chicken baked without the skin.

Food abundance and variety mean that we as consumers need to be smarter in making food decisions. I would never want to see the variety disappear, as it does make the world of food more interesting. As a nutritionist, I find keeping up with new foods and changes in existing foods keeps me very busy. It can be confusing, but it can also be a challenge!

Social pressure to consume more food than our body needs may be stressful. We need to become smarter about handling those situations. To some, the easiest solution is to decrease their social commitments that have food as an integral part. This is an unsatisfactory solution. It leads to resentment and guilt. It does not increase food-decision skills in a social situation. Consider some of the following responses when you are faced with twenty dishes of favorite foods in your favorite company of friends. It's possible to make a social function a positive reflection of your ability to normalize weight for health.

"I'm improving my health! Please make that a small piece of birthday cake as I also want some ice cream. I walked two miles this afternoon so I could attend the party and have cake and ice cream without feeling guilty."

"Christmas is my favorite time of year. I enjoy sharing the company of my friends. I care about my friends and they care about me. Rather than food, may we exchange flowers?"

"I'm excited about seeing this film. The reviews have been outstanding. Diet soda and unbuttered popcorn, please."

"It was thoughtful of you to bring in doughnuts for everyone this morning. Let's go for a walk during our lunch break so I can eat one without feeling guilty."

"Would you like to go to the beach on Saturday? I just bought a new swimsuit to match my new figure!"

Healthy food decisions lead to long-term benefits. High blood pressure is known as the silent killer. In some ways, healthy food decisions are just as silent. It will take time for you to experience all of the benefits. It's not an instant process. Only one or two days of making changes lead to more anger and frustration than to health benefits. Make a ten-week commitment. This will be enough time to experience some of the many benefits.

My hope is that you confidently make food decisions that promote health. What you eat and drink affects the way you feel.

Small Changes Make Big Differences

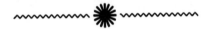

The purpose of this chapter is to illustrate how making small changes in your food pattern can make big differences over time. It will help you identify specific activities and foods that can be modified for long-term benefits. The chapter is not a list of "good behaviors" and "bad behaviors." It's up to you to negotiate acceptable modifications. Your health is your responsibility.

The first time my patients come to see me they are expecting the magical "diet sheet." They soon discover that time will be spent identifying single changes that can make big differences over time. Perhaps you can identify with the "soda addict," "business drinker," or "fast-food luncher."

Many people have a soda habit. "No, I don't eat breakfast. I have a soda." Do you start your day with a sugar fix? A twelve-ounce can of sweetened soda contains the equivalent of ten packages (⅕ cup) of sugar. This equals 160 calories. One can per day for a year adds up to 58,400 calories. This equals seventeen pounds of body fat per year!

Making a change is a deliberate action. There are alternatives to the soda habit. Substitute an artificially sweetened soda. Or drink half the amount of regular soda you normally consume. Drink water. I have talked to many people who are part of a family that easily consumes six sodas each day at a cost of $900 per year! Save the money for new clothes, books, music, travel, flowers, or anything else you enjoy.

The pressure is on the business drinker. A business decision is casually being formulated and finalized in a bar. Perhaps you are getting to know a new client. The drinks flow!

There are alternatives to using a bar to finalize a business decision. Ask the client if he or she would be willing to walk for fifteen minutes. Tell them that you consider it less distracting. A fifteen-minute walk burns 100 calories. In addition, it's time during which you will not be drinking. The walk in combination with less drinking equals 300 fewer calories. If you do this three times per week, it will equal 900 fewer calories. Over a year, this will equal a weight loss of thirteen pounds!

If you normally have four drinks per social visit to the bar, substitute a drink with a low-calorie beverage. Each substitution equals 200 to 300 calories. If you make the substitution three times per week, you will lose eleven pounds in a year.

Do you know a fast-food luncher? "Every day for the last twelve years I've been eating a burger, fries, and a milkshake for lunch. There cannot possibly be an acceptable alternative to that!"

Fast-food restaurants offer a wide variety of nutritious foods that can be incorporated into your food pattern. However, keep the food-decision process in mind. Select foods that are part of the basic four food groups. Reduce portions. Be aware of the effect of food preparation on the calorie and sodium contents of foods. Study the Heart Factors and fat content of fast foods as shown in the chapter on Fast Foods on page 167.

Consider the beef burgers at McDonald's. A hamburger

has 254 calories. A cheeseburger has 306 calories. A Quarter Pounder has 421 calories. A Quarter Pounder with cheese has 522 calories. A Big Mac has 566 calories. A McDLT has 680 calories. Be informed. It all adds up!

A chocolate milkshake has 381 calories. Substitute a soft-serve ice cream cone that contains 190 calories. This equals 570 fewer calories per week if you make the substitution three times a week. Over a year, the substitution will equal a weight loss of nine pounds!

Walk to the fast-food restaurant. One mile equals 100 calories.

Consciously make food decisions rather than follow a food pattern that has not worked to optimize your health. Food habits evolve out of convenience and preference. Do not judge habits or individual foods as either "good" or "bad." Guilt has very little to do with making informed food decisions. Be creative in finding acceptable alternatives that will make big differences over time.

Small Changes Make Big Differences

	Calories		
	High	*Low*	*Saved*
BEVERAGES:			
black coffee for cream & sugar	100	0	100
daiquiri (4 oz) for eggnog	335	120	215
diet soda (12-oz can) for regular	160	5	155
dry wine (4 oz) for sweet	175	145	30
"lite" beer (12-oz can) for regular	175	100	75
skim milk (8 oz) for whole	165	80	85
SNACKS:			
grapes (1 cup) for chocolate (1 oz)	145	65	80
plain popcorn (2 cups) for candied	270	110	160
small pretzels (10) for potato chips	115	35	80
soybean nuts (1 oz) for peanuts	170	125	45
MEATS:			
baked chicken (no skin) for fried	400	200	200
ham (3 oz) for pork sausage	405	200	205
poached eggs (2) for fried	220	160	60
water-packed tuna (3 oz) for oil-packed	180	95	85
VEGETABLES:			
asparagus (1 cup) for lima beans	160	30	130
green beans (1 cup) for baked beans	320	30	190
mashed potatoes (1 cup) for fried	480	245	235
DESSERTS:			
ice milk (4 oz) for ice cream	350	185	165
low-calorie pudding (4 oz) for regular	180	65	115
plain doughnut (1) for jelly-filled	225	125	100
MISCELLANEOUS:			
apple butter on toast for butter	90	15	75
clear soup (1 cup) for creamed soup	210	110	100
low-calorie dressing (1 tbsp) for regular	70	20	50

How many calories can you save today?

The Grocery Store

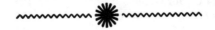

The trip to the grocery store begins in the kitchen. Food in the refrigerator, freezer, or kitchen cabinet is the food that will eventually become a part of your diet.

The United States is a country of many choices. Walking by a grocery store the other day, I noticed a sign that said there were ten thousand reasons to shop there. Most grocery stores have more than five thousand different food items to select from. Making food decisions for health rapidly becomes confusing when you consider all the possibilities. There is so much information!

Begin simply. Select foods that you enjoy and that will provide essential nutrients. It is easy to shop by the basic four food groups: fruits and vegetables, dairy products, breads and starches, and finally meats. Each food group is packed with important nutrients for health. To exclude a food group is to exclude nutrients essential for health. If you just consumed foods listed in the "diet sheet," your weekly list would include:

118

I. Fruits and Vegetables:

banana (7 per week)

fruit (14 per week): apple, blueberries, cantaloupe, grapefruit, pear, orange, peach, pineapple, tangerine, and strawberries

salad, 1½ cups (7 per week): beets, bell peppers, celery, carrots, cucumbers, lettuce, mushrooms, onion, tomatoes, squash, and zucchini

vegetable, 1 cup (7 per week): asparagus, broccoli, cabbage, cauliflower, eggplant, green beans, greens, and spinach

II. Breads and Starches:

cereal (7 per week): shredded wheat, All-Bran, Grape-nuts, Cream of Wheat, and Nutri-Grain

starchy vegetable, ½ cup (3 per week): corn, potatoes, peas

bread (4 per week): bread, dinner roll, rice, grits

III. Meats:

tuna or chicken, ½ cup (3 per week)

chicken, 4 oz (3 per week)

fish, 4 oz (3 per week)

pork chop (1 per week)

IV. Dairy Products:

skim milk, 1 cup (7 per week)

low-fat cottage cheese, ½ cup (4 per week)

Add additional foods to account for walking or other exercises.

Have a plan when you go to the grocery store. Take an imaginary tour. Often you are welcomed into the store by the week's specials. Perhaps it is the Valentine's Day candy that didn't sell. Calories at half price! What a bargain! Empty calories, even at half price, are *not* a bargain.

Quickly walk to the produce department. Fresh fruits and vegetables are the best thing going. In terms of nutrition, the foods are very low in sodium and fat, and very high in potassium, fiber, and vitamin C. Also, it's hard to get bored with the variety in shape, size, and color. "I don't want to be a rabbit!" Is this your response when you first view salad ingredients? Twenty-four-hour dietary recall data was collected from 11,658 adult Americans in the National Health and Nutrition Examination Survey. It was learned that on a typical day, 40 percent of Americans do not eat a single fruit, and 18 percent eat no vegetables. Your mother would be shocked!

Now that you've loaded up your shopping basket with plenty of fresh fruits and vegetables, you'll walk by a zillion dressings with plenty of salt and fat to cover up the taste. Some people want salads to slide down. Use lemon juice, vinegar, spices, or a dressing that doesn't contain any oil. Try crunchy!

Dressings are often followed by a "diet food" section. Diet foods are expensive and unnecessary. Basic foods work best.

The cookie section is just on your right. Pat yourself on the back as you walk on by. Don't fret. The cookie packages are safely closed. Have you ever noticed how cookies disappear when the package is open? When you've reached some of your goals, you'll be able to incorporate cookies and cakes without feeling guilty. This is best done by purchasing pre-packaged single-portion items.

At this point, you turn left and on your right is quite a large variety of beers. Beer does not contain any fat and is very low in sodium. However, there are still plenty of calories. There are 7 calories per gram of alcohol. Moderation works best. I like to split a "lite" beer with my husband.

It's time to go down the aisles. The first aisle displays pickles, olives, vinegar, ketchup, mustard, etc. It has happened more than once that a patient of mine has stopped using salt and found it much easier to drink pickle juice. The Heart Factor for one large dill pickle is 57! Also, olives are very high in fat! Purchase some vinegar to tenderize meats. It does not contain any salt or fat.

The second aisle displays canned vegetables, fruits, and juice. Canned goods are convenient and economical. There are a few factors to note. First, canned vegetables usually contain 200 to 300 mg of sodium per serving. If you have a choice between eating canned vegetables and not eating vegetables, then eat canned vegetables! When possible, eat fresh or frozen vegetables. It's convenient to use fresh or frozen vegetables because you can prepare the exact amount that you want to eat. Also, it's much more economical to eat fresh or frozen vegetables than to purchase a small can of low-sodium vegetables.

While soups are low in calories, they also tend to be very salty. Make a vegetable soup by starting with canned tomatoes, corn, and/or black-eyed peas, then simply add any fresh vegetables (carrots, onions, green beans, potatoes, etc.) until you get tired of chopping. The flavor becomes more interesting as you add more vegetables. The sodium content of the homemade soup will still be much lower than that of any canned soup.

Make sure that canned fruit is packed in water or its own juice rather than a heavy syrup. Packing fruits in syrup increases calories. Down the aisle you will find juice. I like 100 percent unsweetened juice in individual portions. Juice is low in sodium and fat while it is high in potassium and vitamin C. I usually take a six pack of grapefruit juice in my car. It's convenient and refreshing to have some juice when I drive to work or sit in traffic.

The bread section of the grocery store is next. Bread is good for you. Select whole-grain breads, which are high in fiber. Be selective about what you put on the bread.

Turning left, you find the meat section. Cold cuts are high in salt and fat. Turkey- or poultry-based cold cuts have less fat. As you begin modifying your food pattern select mostly chicken, turkey, and fish. One pork chop a week is fine if you trim off the fat. Meats are low in sodium, high in potassium, and high in protein. Take note of the weight of meats and estimate the number of servings per package. One serving equals three to four ounces.

If you select canned tuna or chicken, make sure it is water-packed. Start dietary changes with fresh fruit as portions are easier to control in addition to the fact that it actually takes more time to eat fresh fruit than to drink a juice. Peanut butter is pretty high in fat and salt. Jams and jellies are deceptively high in calories. Apple butter is a better choice.

At one time cornflakes and oatmeal were the major options for breakfast cereals. Today, choice is much more complicated. Cereals vary significantly in sugar, fiber, and salt content. Start with shredded wheat, since the portion can be easily determined and the cereal is high in fiber, low in salt, and low in sugar. Other reasonable choices are Grapenuts, Wheat Chex, Nutri-Grain, Cream of Wheat, or oatmeal. Read and compare food labels.

Coffee, tea, and condiments are close by the cereals. The caffeine in tea and coffee is probably all right in moderation. Focus on making food decisions to normalize weight. Some of the spices to flavor foods are: cinnamon, chili powder, chives, dill, garlic powder, lemon juice, mustard, onion powder, oregano, parsley, pepper, and vinegar. Experiment! The chapter on recipes will give you a detailed listing of condiments and their many uses.

All oils are pure fat. Naturally the oils do not contain cholesterol, but they certainly contain calories! Walk to the dog-food section. At this point you may be wishing for something as simple as people food. The only food decision would be the amount.

Danger! Walk or run past the snack foods. Chips contain a tremendous amount of salt and fat. No one can realistically eat just one. If you buy it, you eat it! Do not be tempted to purchase any soda with sugar. One can of sweetened soda contains ten packages ($\frac{1}{5}$ cup) of sugar. It is fine to substitute sweet soda with diet soda. But soda tends to represent a lot of money for very little nutrition.

There are many more frozen foods to select. Read labels carefully. Know what you're doing. Don't get the vegetables with all the sauces. Select simple foods. Ice cream is tempting. Perhaps a fruit bar can be a good substitute. Pizza has too much salt and too many calories. You will be able to include all foods in your diet after you reach a normal weight.

Include dairy products. Select skim milk. A lunch might be plain yogurt with fresh fruit. The meal will be high in protein and calcium. Use low-fat cottage cheese. Read labels. Both margarine and butter are solid fat. The breakfast items of eggs, bacon, and sausage are often located next to the dairy products. Egg whites or egg substitutes are very low in calories, while egg yolks are high in fat and cholesterol. Bacon and sausage are high in salt and fat. One sausage pattie equals over 200 calories.

You've made it to the checkout! Don't give in to the candy. Give yourself credit for the smart food decisions. You can make the difference because you are in control. Oh, stop by the produce section and buy yourself a few flowers.

Enjoy the grocery store. It's an opportunity to think actively about food. You will succeed if you have a plan in mind.

Exercise

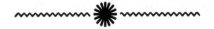

My dad spent his sixty-seventh birthday climbing to the base camp at Mount Everest. My brothers, sisters, and I look forward to the day when we can become as fit as Dad! Consult your doctor before you begin an exercise program.

It is difficult to assess the relationship between exercise and incidence of coronary heart disease. Physical activity, unlike the other risk factors of high blood pressure, high serum cholesterol, and cigarette smoking, lacks standard assessment methods.

However, it is estimated that approximately 59 percent of Americans do not engage in any regular physical activity. The definition of regular physical activity is three or more times per week for at least twenty minutes each time. One hour a week does not sound like a lot of exercise, but if it is of adequate intensity, it will maintain fitness.

Exercise is fundamental to health. Exercise keeps you strong. Exercise burns calories. Special equipment or scheduling of your time is not essential. It is easy to make exercise a part of your day. The opportunities are everywhere!

Increase exercise by walking up the stairs. It may sound trite but stairs are just a series of steps. You may be thinking,

"Where can I find the stairs?" All buildings have them for safety reasons. Know where the stairs are located in the unlikely but possible event of a fire. For safety—take time to find the stairs in any building you are in.

"The elevator is here! It's easier!" But it's rare for the elevator door to open the moment you appear. Taking an elevator often means standing and waiting. "I've walked half a flight of stairs. My heart is pounding." The first time up the stairs will be the hardest. Use good judgment. Fitness improves with time. Later, you will be amused to discover that locating the stairs may have been the hardest part!

Your destination is the sixth floor. You haven't exercised in a long time. Don't charge up six flights and be overly exhausted at the top. Climb one flight. Rest. Climb the second flight. Take the elevator the rest of the way. As you become fit, the distance will become much easier. Recognize stair climbing as an opportunity to include exercise into your day sensibly. It will become easier to do as your strength increases, your weight decreases, and your confidence increases. Go down the stairs too. It's very easy.

Driving a car has replaced much walking. The automobile has greatly increased our mobility. We see and do much more than if we were limited to walking alone. Do simple things to increase exercise. Park the car on the opposite side of the parking lot. There is little competition for that space. The time to walk the extra steps is very little.

Where do you live, work, play, and shop? Are there times when you could walk to the corner store? Looking for a place to park may take more time than walking. However, there are times when walking isn't practical. I live six miles from my office and it's not realistic to walk to work. Nevertheless, I can park the car a half mile away. Walking is easy when you make it a habit. Use a stopwatch for a few days to discover how much time you spend walking. Use your imagination!

There are so many step savers in our lives that we may think that we must drive to a gym to put the steps back in.

This is ironic because many forms of exercise are available. While attending gym classes can be enjoyable for comradeship, I primarily encourage you to identify the step savers during the day that can be replaced by your steps. Make walking a habit today.

Calories are a measurement of the amount of energy that comes from food. Exercise requires energy. The intensity of the exercise increases or decreases the number of calories burned. Walking quickly burns more calories than walking slowly. The amount of energy burned varies when you play tennis. A game of singles would probably be more strenuous than a doubles game. Certainly, the energy burned varies with the golfer who drives a cart and the golfer who walks and carries a bag.

Your body weight also changes the amount of energy burned. It requires more energy to carry a body that weighs 240 pounds up ten flights of stairs than to carry a body that weighs 120 pounds.

You may be familiar with tables that tell you how many calories are burned doing specific activities for a specific amount of time. The following table shows the number of calories that are burned if you walk a mile at varied rates. The more you weigh, the more calories you will burn.

Calories Burned per Mile of Walking

Rate	100 Lb	120 Lb	140 Lb	160 Lb	200 Lb
2.0 mph	43	51	55	60	68
2.5 mph	45	52	57	62	72
3.0 mph	47	54	59	64	76
3.5 mph	49	56	61	65	78
4.0 mph	51	57	62	69	82

If you weigh 120 pounds, you will burn 54 calories for every mile walked at the rate of three miles per hour.

Calories Burned per Minutes of Activity

Activity	Cal/Min	10 Min	20 Min	30 Min	40 Min
archery	3.4	34	68	102	136
backpacking	8.8	88	176	264	352
badminton	7.0	70	140	210	280
basketball	8.0	80	160	240	320
bicycling	6.0	60	120	180	240
bowling	2.7	27	54	81	108
calisthenics	6.0	60	120	180	240
canoeing	6.0	60	120	180	240
dancing	5.1	51	102	153	204
fishing, boat	2.7	27	54	81	108
fishing, stream	5.7	57	114	171	228
football—touch	8.8	88	176	264	352
golf—power cart	2.1	21	42	63	84
golf—walking	5.8	58	116	174	232
handball	11.5	115	230	345	460
hiking	5.1	51	102	153	204
horseback riding	6.0	60	120	180	240
mountain climbing	8.0	80	160	240	320
Ping-Pong	3.8	38	76	114	152
racquetball	11.5	115	230	345	460
running					
5.0-min mile	23.5	235	470	705	940
5.5-min mile	20.7	207	414	621	828
6.0-min mile	18.6	186	372	558	744
7.5-min mile	14.6	146	292	438	584
8.5-min mile	13.0	130	260	390	520
10.0-min mile	11.0	110	220	330	440
11.0-min mile	9.1	91	182	273	364
running					
12.0 mph	23.5	235	470	705	940
10.9 mph	20.7	207	414	621	828
10.0 mph	18.6	186	372	558	744
8.0 mph	14.6	146	292	438	584
7.0 mph	13.0	130	260	390	520

Calories Burned per Minutes of Activity *continued*

Activity	Cal/Min	10 Min	20 Min	30 Min	40 Min
6.0 mph	11.0	110	220	330	440
5.5 mph	9.1	91	182	273	364
sailing	3.2	32	64	96	128
scuba diving	8.0	80	160	240	320
shuffleboard	2.1	21	42	63	84
skating, ice	8.0	80	160	240	320
skating, roller	8.0	80	160	240	320
skiing					
cross-country	10.2	102	204	306	408
downhill	8.0	80	160	240	320
soccer	9.0	90	180	270	360
softball	4.6	46	92	138	184
squash	11.5	115	230	345	460
stair climbing	6.5	65	130	195	260
swimming	6.5	65	130	195	260
tennis	7.0	70	140	210	280
volleyball	4.6	46	92	138	184
walking					
30-min mile	1.5	15	30	45	60
24-min mile	2.0	20	40	60	80
20-min mile	2.7	27	54	81	108
17-min mile	3.2	32	64	96	128
16-min mile	3.9	39	78	117	156
15-min mile	4.5	45	90	135	180
12-min mile	7.3	73	146	219	292
walking					
2.0 mph	1.5	15	30	45	60
2.5 mph	2.0	20	40	60	80
3.0 mph	2.7	27	54	81	108
3.5 mph	3.2	32	64	96	128
4.0 mph	4.5	45	90	135	180
5.0 mph	7.3	73	146	219	292

Minutes of Activity Equal to Specific Calories

Activity	50	100	150	200	250
archery	14.7	29.4	44.1	58.8	73.5
backpacking	5.7	11.4	17.0	22.7	28.4
badminton	7.1	14.3	21.4	28.6	35.7
basketball	6.3	12.5	18.8	25.0	31.3
bicycling	8.3	16.7	25.0	33.3	41.7
bowling	18.5	37.0	55.6	74.1	92.6
calisthenics	8.3	16.7	25.0	33.3	41.7
canoeing	8.3	16.7	25.0	33.3	41.7
dancing	9.8	19.6	29.4	39.2	49.0
fishing, boat	18.5	37.0	55.6	74.1	92.6
fishing, stream	8.8	17.5	26.3	35.1	43.9
football—touch	5.7	11.4	17.0	22.7	28.4
golf—power cart	23.8	47.6	71.4	95.2	119.0
golf—walking	8.6	17.2	25.9	34.5	43.1
handball	4.3	8.7	13.0	17.4	21.7
hiking	9.8	19.6	29.4	39.2	49.0
horseback riding	8.3	16.7	25.0	33.3	41.7
mountain climbing	6.3	12.5	18.8	25.0	31.3
Ping-Pong	13.2	26.3	39.5	52.6	65.8
racquetball	4.3	8.7	13.0	17.4	21.7
running					
5.0-min mile	2.1	4.3	6.4	8.5	10.6
5.5-min mile	2.4	4.8	7.2	9.7	12.1
6.0-min mile	2.7	5.4	8.1	10.8	13.4
7.5-min mile	3.4	6.8	10.3	13.7	17.1
8.5-min mile	3.8	7.7	11.5	15.4	19.2
10.0-min mile	4.5	9.1	13.6	18.2	22.7
11.0-min mile	5.5	11.0	16.5	22.0	27.5
running					
12.0 mph	2.1	4.3	6.4	8.5	10.6
10.9 mph	2.4	4.8	7.2	9.7	12.1
10.0 mph	2.7	5.4	8.1	10.8	13.4
8.0 mph	3.4	6.8	10.3	13.7	17.1
7.0 mph	3.8	7.7	11.5	15.4	19.2

Minutes of Activity Equal to Specific Calories *continued*

Activity	50	100	150	200	250
6.0 mph	4.5	9.1	13.6	18.2	22.7
5.5 mph	5.5	11.0	16.5	22.0	27.5
sailing	15.6	31.3	46.9	62.5	78.1
scuba diving	6.3	12.5	18.8	25.0	31.3
shuffleboard	23.8	47.6	71.4	95.2	119.0
skating, ice	6.3	12.5	18.8	25.0	31.3
skating, roller	6.3	12.5	18.8	25.0	31.3
skiing					
cross-country	4.9	9.8	14.7	19.6	24.5
downhill	6.3	12.5	18.8	25.0	31.3
soccer	5.6	11.1	16.7	22.2	27.8
softball	10.9	21.7	32.6	43.5	54.3
squash	4.3	8.7	13.0	17.4	21.7
stair climbing	7.7	15.4	23.1	30.8	38.5
swimming	7.7	15.4	23.1	30.8	38.5
tennis	7.1	14.3	21.4	28.6	35.7
volleyball	10.9	21.7	32.6	43.5	54.3
walking					
30-min mile	33.3	66.7	100.0	133.3	166.7
24-min mile	25.0	50.0	75.0	100.0	125.0
20-min mile	18.5	37.0	55.6	74.1	92.6
17-min mile	15.6	31.3	46.9	62.5	78.1
16-min mile	12.8	25.6	38.5	51.3	64.1
15-min mile	11.1	22.2	33.3	44.4	55.6
12-min mile	6.8	13.7	20.5	27.4	34.2
walking					
2.0 mph	33.3	66.7	100.0	133.3	166.7
2.5 mph	25.0	50.0	75.0	100.0	125.0
3.0 mph	18.5	37.0	55.6	74.1	92.6
3.5 mph	15.6	31.3	46.9	62.5	78.1
4.0 mph	11.1	22.2	33.3	44.4	55.6
5.0 mph	6.8	13.7	20.5	27.4	34.2

Food and Walking Exchange

Foods equal to walking one mile:

beer, "lite"	12 oz
butter	1 tbsp
cream cheese	1 oz
dressing	2 tbsp
fig bars	2
jelly beans	15
light cream	3 tbsp
mayonnaise	1 tbsp
peanut butter	1 tbsp
popcorn	2 cups
pretzels	20 rings
Swiss cheese	1 oz
sherbet	½ cup
wine, dry	4 oz

Foods equal to walking one and a half miles:

avocado	½
bacon	2 slices
beer, regular	12 oz
chocolate bar	1 oz
Coke	12 oz
corn chips	1 oz
doughnut, plain	1
eggs, poached	2
English muffin	1
ice milk	½ cup
martini	3½ oz
Mounds	1 oz
potato chips	1 oz
Snickers	1 oz
wine, sweet	4 oz

Foods equal to walking two miles:

brownie	1½ oz
danish	1
ice cream	½ cup

Food and Walking Exchange *continued*

Foods equal to walking two miles:	
nuts	1 oz
substitute red for white meat	3 oz

Foods equal to walking three miles:	
apple pie	⅛
Twinkies	2

Foods equal to walking four miles:	
nuts	2 oz
pecan pie	⅛

Never exchange foods before walking. If you like, save the walking credits for later. Exchange foods for walking only after the walk is completed!

The Hungries

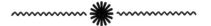

B eware! You have just been attacked by the hungries! It's as predictable as dust under the bed. It can happen when you are reading, watching television, shopping, driving past fast-food restaurants, cooking, visiting with friends, sleeping, or perhaps just after eating a well-balanced meal.

The hungries come in the form of "I want" or "I think I want." Food solves the "I want" attack while it will not solve the "I think I want" attack. When attacked by a hungry, we immediately think that it must be the "I want" variety. The hungries can be very foxy. Think about it a little longer and determine accurately if you have been attacked by "I want" or "I think I want." The following examples will help you decide which one it is.

You and a friend, who has also been struck by the determination to normalize weight, are out for a walk. Both of you are justly proud of yourselves. There have been so many excuses, but today you decide to change. You happen to walk by a doughnut shop. Looks pretty good in there. Your friend says, "Let's just go in and see what happens." The hungries have attacked! It is just one of many "I think I want" attacks.

You're busy and you skip lunch and your afternoon fruit snack. Then when you're driving home, the hungries attack. This time they are the "I want" variety. You are very hungry because you haven't eaten all day. A fast-food order of fries would just hit the spot. This is a good time to have a six-pack of juice in the car. Drink some juice to satisfy the hungry attack until you can have a balanced, low-fat meal. In this case food is the solution.

It's seven in the evening. You normally eat at six. You walk into the house and begin to fix dinner. It takes ten minutes to prepare your nutritious meal and another five minutes to eat it. Then the hungries attack. This time they are the "I think I want" variety. You've eaten but you haven't allowed the twenty minutes necessary for the food to be digested and absorbed to defeat the hungries.

The hungries have no mercy. Everyone falls victim from time to time. First, know that you are being attacked. Second, determine the type of attack. Is it an "I want" attack or is it an "I think I want" attack? Food is the solution to "I want," while diversion is the solution to "I think I want." To divert your attention, it might help to have rice paper pages handy that could be eaten during an attack. Each page would deliciously describe a homemade chocolate chip cookie topped with a pecan; a pizza with extra olives, pepperoni, and cheese; a bacon, lettuce, and tomato sandwich with real mayonnaise; a bag of potato chips that says "You can't eat just one"; and finally, an ice cream sundae with butterscotch syrup, whipped cream, and a cherry on top. Imagine. If you eat this page, you save 894 calories, or 0.26 pounds. The problem with this idea is that the pages would quickly disappear and you need the information!

Recipes

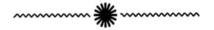

F ood combinations greatly increase variety in flavor, texture, and taste. After reading this chapter you will be able to calculate the nutrient content of your favorite recipes skillfully. Through this you will be able to make simple recipe modifications that improve your nutrition.

Food tables using household measurements are provided to facilitate the calculation of the calories, fat content, and Heart Factor of baked products. Tables are also provided to calculate the sodium and potassium contents individually.

Follow the sample recipe shown below by adding the calories for each ingredient in a basic white bread recipe. The table is similar to a mileage table found on maps. Rather than matching two cities to find the distance, match the portion with the ingredient to determine the calorie content of the specific portion.

Calorie Content of Foods Used in Baking

Food	1 Tbsp	¼ Cup	⅓ Cup	½ Cup	⅔ Cup	¾ Cup	1 Cup
2% fat milk	8	30	40	61	81	91	121
vegetable oil	120	480	640	960	1280	1440	1920
white sugar	50	199	265	398	531	597	796
all-purpose flour	25	100	133	200	267	300	400

	¼ tsp	½ tsp	1 tsp	1 tbsp
salt	0	0	0	0
yeast	2	4	8	23

WHITE BREAD—*1 Loaf (12 Servings)*

		Calories
2% fat milk	*1 cup*	*121*
yeast	*1 tbsp*	*23*
salt	*1 tsp*	*0*
vegetable oil	*1 tbsp*	*120*
white sugar	*2 tbsp*	*100*
all-purpose flour	*3 cups*	*+1200*
	RECIPE	*1564*

Divide the calorie content of the recipe by the number of servings to determine the calorie content of an individual serving.

$$\frac{1564 \text{ recipe calories}}{12 \text{ servings}} = 130 \text{ calories per serving}$$

The Heart Factor Food Plan means paying attention to fat, sodium, and potassium. Use the tables to determine the fat content of the recipe. To simplify the sodium and potassium calculations, determine the Heart Factor of the recipe. Remember that the Heart Factor equals the milliequivalent of sodium minus the milliequivalent of potassium. A high Heart Factor equals high sodium, which equals high blood pressure.

Fat (Grams) in Foods Used in Baking

Food	1 Tbsp	¼ Cup	⅓ Cup	½ Cup	⅔ Cup	¾ Cup	1 Cup
2% fat milk	0	1	2	2	3	4	5
vegetable oil	14	56	74	111	148	166	222
white sugar	0	0	0	0	0	0	0
all-purpose flour	0	0	0	1	1	1	1

	¼ tsp	½ tsp	1 tsp	1 tbsp
salt	0	0	0	0
yeast	0	0	0	0

Heart Factor of Foods Used in Baking

Food	1 Tbsp	¼ Cup	⅓ Cup	½ Cup	⅔ Cup	¾ Cup	1 Cup
2% fat milk	0	−1	−1	−2	−3	−3	−4
vegetable oil	0	0	0	0	0	0	0
white sugar	0	0	0	0	0	0	0
all-purpose flour	0	−1	−1	−1	−2	−2	−3

	¼ tsp	½ tsp	1 tsp	1 tbsp
salt	24	47	94	282
yeast	0	−1	−1	−4

WHITE BREAD—*1 Loaf (12 Servings)*

		Calories	Fat	HF
2% fat milk	1 cup	121	2	−4
yeast	1 tbsp	23	0	−1
salt	1 tsp	0	0	94
vegetable oil	1 tbsp	120	14	0
white sugar	2 tbsp	100	0	0
all-purpose flour	3 cups	+1200	+3	+−9
	RECIPE	1564	19	80

1 serving = 130 calories = 2 grams of fat = 7 Heart Factor

One serving of white bread contains 2 grams of fat and has a Heart Factor of 7. A pat of margarine would increase the total fat content of 2 grams to 7 grams of fat per serving. Sometimes it is useful to estimate the percent of calories that comes from fat in recipes. Fat should provide no more than 30 to 35 percent of your total calories. The percent of calories from fat can be calculated by multiplying the grams of fat times nine and dividing by the total calories. Multiply this number by 100 to estimate the percent.

% fat = ((grams of fat × 9) / total calories) × 100
% fat = ((19 × 9) ÷ 1564) × 100 = 11% fat

The white bread recipe contains 120 calories from the fat in the vegetable oil. Fat equals 8 percent of the total calories. White bread is very low in fat.

Percent Fat	
0– 15%	= very low
16– 25%	= low
26– 35%	= medium
36– 45%	= high
46–100%	= very high

The white bread recipe can be modified to make whole-wheat bread by changing white flour to a combination of white flour and whole-wheat flour and changing white sugar to molasses.

WHOLE-WHEAT BREAD—*1 Loaf (12 Servings)*

		Calories	Fat	HF
2% fat milk	1 cup	121	2	−4
yeast	1 tbsp	23	0	−1
salt	1 tsp	0	0	94
vegetable oil	1 tbsp	120	14	0
molasses	2 tbsp	96	0	−14
all-purpose flour	1½ cups	600	2	−4
whole-wheat flour	1½ cups	+600	+3	+−9
	RECIPE	1560	21	62

one loaf = 1560 calories = 21 grams of fat = 62 Heart
  Factor
1 serving = 130 calories = 2 grams of fat = 5 Heart
  Factor
% fat = ((21 × 9) ÷ 1560) × 100 = 12% fat = very
  low

The Heart Factor of whole-wheat bread is less than that
of white bread because whole-wheat flour and molasses are
higher in potassium. The positive effects of the high-potassium ingredients reduce the negative effects of the high-sodium ingredients.

The Heart Factor of all foods can be reduced by deleting
or reducing salt. Consider the impact this has on the Heart
Factor of the white bread.

WHITE BREAD—*1 Loaf (12 Servings)*

		Calories	Fat	HF
2% fat milk	1 cup	121	2	−4
yeast	1 tbsp	23	0	−1
vegetable oil	1 tbsp	120	14	0
white sugar	2 tbsp	100	0	0
all-purpose flour	3 cups	+1200	+3	+−9
	RECIPE	1564	19	−14

*1 serving = 130 calories = 2 grams of fat = −1
   Heart Factor*
*% fat = ((19 × 9) ÷ 1564) × 100 = 11% fat =
   very low*

Biscuits differ from bread in that the fat content is much higher. The Heart Factor is increased because self-rising flour contains salt for flavor and baking powder for leavening.

BISCUITS—*12 Servings*

		Calories	Fat	HF
2% fat milk	1 cup	121	5	−4
shortening	⅓ cup	554	62	0
self-rising flour	2¼ cups	+981	+2	+113
	RECIPE	1656	69	109

*1 serving = 138 calories = 6 grams of fat = 9 Heart
   Factor*
% fat = ((69 × 9) ÷ 1656) × 100 = 38% fat = high

My mother was English, so it was common in our house to have rock cakes for tea. Rock cakes are a cross between a biscuit and cake.

ROCK CAKES—*20 Servings*

		Calories	Fat	HF
margarine	½ cup	831	92	48
white sugar	⅔ cup	531	0	0
raisins	⅔ cup	300	0	−17
nutmeg	1 tsp*			
self-rising flour	2½ cups	1090	3	125
2% fat milk	½ cup	61	2	12
egg	1	+79	+6	+1
	RECIPE	2892	103	169

1 serving = 145 calories = 5 grams of fat = 8 Heart Factor

% fat = ((97 × 9) ÷ 2892) × 100 = 30% fat = medium

---

*Flavorings and spices do not contribute significantly to calorie, fat, and HF calculations.

OATMEAL RAISIN COOKIES—*30 Servings*

		Calories	Fat	HF
white sugar	½ cup	398	0	0
brown sugar	½ cup	434	0	−6
margarine	½ cup	831	92	48
egg	1	79	6	1
vanilla	1 tsp*			
baking powder	½ tsp	0	0	10
baking soda	½ tsp	0	0	18
cinnamon	1 tsp*			
all-purpose flour	1 cup	400	1	−3
2% fat milk	2 tbsp	16	0	0
oatmeal	1 cup	333	6	−8
raisins	½ cup	+225	+0	+−13
	RECIPE	2716	105	47

1 serving = 91 calories = 4 grams of fat = 2 Heart
  Factor
% fat = ((105 × 9) ÷ 2716) × 100 = 35% fat =
  medium

*Flavorings and spices do not contribute significantly to calorie, fat, and HF calculations.

ROLLED ALMOND COOKIES—*25 Servings*

		Calories	Fat	HF
margarine	½ cup	831	92	48
white sugar	¾ cup	597	0	0
egg	1	79	6	1
almond extract	1 tsp*			
baking powder	1½ tsp	0	0	29
salt	¼ tsp	0	0	24
all-purpose flour	2 cups	800	2	−6
2% fat milk	1 tbsp	+9	+0	+0
	RECIPE	2316	100	96

1 serving = 93 calories = 4 grams of fat = 4 Heart
  Factor
% fat = ((100 × 9) ÷ 2316) × 100 = 39% fat =
  high

*Flavorings and spices do not contribute significantly to calorie, fat, and HF calculations.

YELLOW CAKE—*12 Servings*

		Calories	Fat	HF
eggs	2	158	11	2
white sugar	1 cup	796	0	0
margarine	½ cup	831	92	48
vanilla	1 tsp*			
2% fat milk	½ cup	61	2	−2
self-rising flour	2 cups	+872	+2	+100
	RECIPE	2718	107	148

1 serving = 227 calories = 9 grams of fat = 12
Heart Factor
% fat = ((107 × 9) ÷ 2718) × 100 = 35% fat =
medium

POUND CAKE—*16 Servings*

		Calories	Fat	HF
eggs	4	316	22	4
white sugar	1 cup	796	0	0
margarine	1 cup	1662	185	97
lemon juice	1 tbsp*			
baking powder	1 tsp	0	0	19
all-purpose flour	2 cups	+800	+2	+−6
	RECIPE	3574	209	114

1 serving = 223 calories = 13 grams of fat = 7 Heart
Factor
% fat = ((209 × 9) ÷ 3574) × 100 = 53% fat =
very high

---

*Flavorings and spices do not contribute significantly to calorie, fat, and HF calculations.

Reduce fat by substituting "lite" margarine for regular margarine. In my kitchen I use stick margarine versus tub margarine. Tub margarine does not work well in baking.

POUND CAKE—*16 Servings*

		Calories	*Fat*	*HF*
eggs	*4*	*316*	*22*	*4*
white sugar	*1 cup*	*796*	*0*	*0*
margarine, "lite"	*1 cup*	*1247*	*139*	*90*
lemon juice	*1 tbsp**			
baking powder	*1 tsp*	*0*	*0*	*19*
all-purpose flour	*2 cups*	*+800*	*+2*	*+ −6*
	RECIPE	*3159*	*163*	*107*

*1 serving = 197 calories = 10 grams of fat = 7 Heart
  Factor*
*% fat = ((163 × 9) ÷ 3159) × 100 = 46% fat =
  very high*

---

*Flavorings and spices do not contribute significantly to calorie, fat, and HF calculations.

ANGEL FOOD CAKE—*12 Servings*

		Calories	Fat	HF
vanilla extract	*1 tsp**			
cream of tartar	*1½ tsp**			
egg whites	12	192	0	0
cake flour	*1 cup*	364	1	−2
white sugar	¾ *cup*	513	0	0
powdered sugar	¾ *cup*	+597	+0	+0
	RECIPE	*1666*	*1*	*−2*

*1 serving = 139 calories = 0 grams of fat = 0 Heart
   Factor*
% fat = ((1 × 9) ÷ 1666) × 100 = 0% fat

Gingerbread is a cake that uses molasses for sweetening.
Ginger and cinnamon are added for flavor.

---

*Flavorings and spices do not contribute significantly to calorie, fat, and HF calcu-
lations.

GINGERBREAD—*12 Servings*

		Calories	Fat	HF
eggs	1	79	6	1
vegetable oil	⅓ cup	640	71	0
sugar	½ cup	398	0	0
molasses	½ cup	384	0	−59
baking soda	1 tsp	0	0	36
ginger	1 tsp*			
cinnamon	½ tsp*			
boiling water	½ cup	0	0	0
all-purpose flour	1½ cups	+600	+2	+−4
	RECIPE	2101	79	−16

1 serving = 175 calories = 7 grams of fat = −1 Heart
  Factor

% fat = ((79 × 9) ÷ 2101) × 100 = 34% fat =
  medium

*Flavorings and spices do not contribute significantly to calorie, fat, and HF calcu-
lations.

RAISIN GINGERBREAD—*16 Servings*

		Calories	Fat	HF
eggs	*1*	*79*	*6*	*1*
vegetable oil	*⅓ cup*	*640*	*71*	*0*
sugar	*½ cup*	*398*	*0*	*0*
molasses	*½ cup*	*384*	*0*	*−59*
raisins	*1 cup*	*450*	*0*	*−26*
baking soda	*1 tsp*	*0*	*0*	*36*
ginger	*1 tsp**			
cinnamon	*½ tsp**			
boiling water	*½ cup*	*0*	*0*	*0*
all-purpose flour	*1½ cups*	*+600*	*+2*	*+−4*
	RECIPE	*2551*	*79*	*−52*

1 serving = 159 calories = 7 grams of fat = −3 Heart Factor

% fat = ((79 × 9) ÷ 2551) × 100 = 28% fat = medium

---

*Flavorings and spices do not contribute significantly to calorie, fat, and HF calculations.

Weight (Grams) of Foods Used in Baking

Food	1 Tbsp	¼ Cup	⅓ Cup	½ Cup	⅔ Cup	¾ Cup	1 Cup
GRAIN							
all-purpose flour	7	28	37	56	75	84	112
cake flour	6	25	33	50	67	75	100
cornmeal	9	37	50	75	99	112	149
oatmeal	5	21	28	42	56	63	84
rye flour	7	28	37	56	75	84	112
self-rising flour	7	28	37	56	75	84	112
whole-wheat flour	8	30	40	60	80	90	120
DAIRY							
buttermilk	15	61	82	123	163	184	245
evaporated milk	16	64	85	128	171	192	256
skim milk	15	62	82	123	164	185	246
2% fat milk	15	61	81	122	163	183	244
whole milk	15	61	81	122	163	183	244
SWEETS							
brown sugar	14	56	75	112	149	168	224
chocolate chips	11	42	56	84	112	126	168
coconut, fresh	6	24	32	48	64	72	96
coconut, sweet	5	21	28	42	56	63	84
corn syrup	20	80	107	160	213	240	320
honey	20	80	107	160	213	240	320
molasses	20	80	107	160	213	240	320
powdered sugar	11	45	59	89	119	134	178
raisins	9	38	50	75	100	113	150
white sugar	13	50	67	100	133	150	200
FATS							
margarine	14	57	76	114	152	171	228
margarine, "lite"	9	35	46	69	92	104	139
margarine, unsalted	14	57	76	114	152	171	228
peanut butter	16	64	85	128	171	192	256
shortening	14	57	76	114	152	171	228

Weight (Grams) of Foods Used in Baking *continued*

Food	1 Tbsp	¼ Cup	⅓ Cup	½ Cup	⅔ Cup	¾ Cup	1 Cup
vegetable oil	14	56	75	112	149	168	224
walnuts	8	32	43	64	85	96	128

MISCELLANEOUS	¼ tsp	½ tsp	1 tsp	1 tbsp			
baking powder	1	2	3	9			
baking soda	1	2	3	9			
cocoa powder	1	2	3	7			
salt	1	3	6	18			
salt, "lite"	1	3	6	18			
yeast	2	4	8	23			

EGGS	1	2	3	4	5	6	
egg white	33	66	99	132	165	198	
egg yolk	17	34	51	68	85	102	
whole egg	50	100	150	200	250	300	

Calories in Foods Used in Baking

Food	1 Tbsp	¼ Cup	⅓ Cup	½ Cup	⅔ Cup	¾ Cup	1 Cup
GRAIN							
all-purpose flour	25	100	133	200	267	300	400
cake flour	23	91	121	182	243	273	364
cornmeal	34	136	181	272	363	408	544
oatmeal	21	83	111	167	222	250	333
rye flour	25	98	131	196	261	294	392
self-rising flour	27	109	145	218	291	327	436
whole-wheat flour	25	100	133	200	267	300	400
DAIRY							
buttermilk	6	25	33	50	66	74	99
evaporated milk	19	75	100	150	200	225	300
skim milk	6	22	30	45	59	67	89
2% fat milk	8	30	40	61	81	91	121
whole milk	9	38	50	75	100	113	150
SWEETS							
brown sugar	54	217	289	434	579	651	868
chocolate chips	55	218	291	436	581	654	872
coconut, fresh	22	87	116	174	232	261	348
coconut, sweet	25	101	135	203	270	304	405
corn syrup	59	237	316	474	631	710	947
honey	61	245	327	490	653	735	980
molasses	48	192	256	384	512	576	768
powdered sugar	43	171	228	342	456	513	684
raisins	28	113	150	225	300	338	450
white sugar	50	199	265	398	531	597	796
FATS							
margarine	104	416	554	831	1108	1247	1662
margarine, "lite"	78	312	416	623	831	935	1247
margarine, unsalted	104	416	554	831	1108	1247	1662
peanut butter	92	369	492	738	983	1106	1475
shortening	104	416	554	831	1108	1247	1662

Calories in Foods Used in Baking *continued*

Food	1 Tbsp	¼ Cup	⅓ Cup	½ Cup	⅔ Cup	¾ Cup	1 Cup
vegetable oil	120	480	640	960	1280	1440	1920
walnuts	49	196	261	392	523	588	784

MISCELLANEOUS	¼ tsp	½ tsp	1 tsp	1 tbsp			
baking powder	0	0	0	0			
baking soda	0	0	0	0			
cocoa powder	2	4	7	22			
salt	0	0	0	0			
salt, "lite"	0	0	0	0			
yeast	2	4	8	23			

EGGS	1	2	3	4	5	6	
egg white	16	32	48	64	80	96	
egg yolk	65	126	189	252	315	378	
whole egg	79	158	237	316	395	474	

Fat (Grams) in Foods Used in Baking

Food	1 Tbsp	¼ Cup	⅓ Cup	½ Cup	⅔ Cup	¾ Cup	1 Cup
GRAIN							
all-purpose flour	0	0	0	1	1	1	1
cake flour	0	0	0	1	1	1	1
cornmeal	0	1	1	1	2	2	3
oatmeal	0	2	2	3	4	5	6
rye flour	0	1	1	1	1	1	2
self-rising flour	0	0	0	1	1	1	1
whole-wheat flour	0	1	1	1	2	2	2
DAIRY							
buttermilk	0	0	0	0	0	0	0
evaporated milk	1	5	6	10	13	14	19
skim milk	0	0	0	0	0	0	0
2% fat milk	0	1	2	2	3	4	5
whole milk	1	3	4	6	8	9	12
SWEETS							
brown sugar	0	0	0	0	0	0	0
chocolate chips	3	12	16	24	33	37	49
coconut, fresh	2	8	11	16	22	25	33
coconut, sweet	2	7	9	14	18	21	28
corn syrup	0	0	0	0	0	0	0
honey	0	0	0	0	0	0	0
molasses	0	0	0	0	0	0	0
powdered sugar	0	0	0	0	0	0	0
raisins	0	0	0	0	0	0	0
FATS							
margarine	12	46	62	92	123	139	185
margarine, "lite"	5	22	29	43	58	65	87
margarine, unsalted	12	46	62	92	123	139	185
peanut butter	8	32	42	63	84	95	126
shortening	12	46	62	92	123	139	185

Fat (Grams) in Foods Used in Baking *continued*

Food	1 Tbsp	¼ Cup	⅓ Cup	½ Cup	⅔ Cup	¾ Cup	1 Cup
vegetable oil	13	53	71	107	142	160	213
walnuts	5	21	28	41	55	62	83

MISCELLANEOUS	¼ tsp	½ tsp	1 tsp	1 tbsp
baking powder	0	0	0	0
baking soda	0	0	0	0
cocoa powder	0	0	0	1
salt	0	0	0	0
salt, "lite"	0	0	0	0
yeast	0	0	0	0

EGGS	1	2	3	4	5
egg white	0	0	0	0	0
egg yolk	6	11	17	22	28
whole egg	6	11	17	22	28

Heart Factor of Foods Used in Baking

Food	1 Tbsp	¼ Cup	⅓ Cup	½ Cup	⅔ Cup	¾ Cup	1 Cup
GRAIN							
all-purpose flour	0	−1	−1	−1	−2	−2	−3
cake flour	0	−1	−1	−1	−1	−2	−2
cornmeal	0	−2	−2	−4	−5	−5	−7
oatmeal	−1	−2	−3	−4	−5	−6	−8
rye flour	0	−2	−2	−3	−4	−4	−6
self-rising flour	3	13	17	25	33	37	50
whole-wheat flour	−1	−3	−4	−6	−8	−8	−11
DAIRY							
buttermilk	0	1	2	3	3	4	5
evaporated milk	0	−2	−3	−4	−5	−6	−8
skim milk	0	−1	−1	−2	−2	−3	−4
2% fat milk	0	−1	−1	−2	−3	−3	−4
whole milk	0	−1	−1	−2	−2	−3	−4
SWEETS							
brown sugar	−1	−3	−4	−6	−7	−8	−11
chocolate chips	−1	−3	−4	−6	−8	−9	−12
coconut, fresh	−1	−5	−6	−9	−12	−14	−18
coconut, sweet	0	1	1	1	2	2	3
corn syrup	0	−2	−2	−3	−4	−4	−6
honey	0	−1	−1	−2	−2	−3	−4
molasses	−7	−29	−39	−59	−78	−88	−117
powdered sugar	0	0	0	0	0	0	0
raisins	−2	−7	−9	−13	−17	−19	−26
white sugar	0	0	0	0	0	0	0
FATS							
margarine	6	24	32	48	64	72	97
margarine, "lite"	6	23	30	45	60	68	90
margarine, unsalted	0	0	0	0	0	0	0
peanut butter	2	6	8	12	16	18	24

Heart Factor of Foods Used in Baking *continued*

Food	1 Tbsp	¼ Cup	⅓ Cup	½ Cup	⅔ Cup	¾ Cup	1 Cup
shortening	0	0	0	0	0	0	0
vegetable oil	0	0	0	0	0	0	0
walnuts	−1	−4	−5	−7	−10	−11	−15

MISCELLANEOUS	¼ tsp	½ tsp	1 tsp	1 tbsp
baking powder	5	10	19	57
baking soda	9	18	36	107
cocoa powder	0	0	1	3
salt	24	47	94	282
salt, "lite"	2	5	10	29
yeast	0	−1	−1	−4

EGGS	1	2	3	4	5
egg white	1	2	3	4	5
egg yolk	0	0	0	0	0
whole egg	1	2	3	4	5

Sodium (mg) in Foods Used in Baking

Food	1 Tbsp	¼ Cup	⅓ Cup	½ Cup	⅔ Cup	¾ Cup	1 Cup
GRAIN							
all-purpose flour	0	1	1	2	2	2	3
cake flour	0	1	1	2	2	2	3
cornmeal	0	2	2	3	4	5	6
oatmeal	0	1	1	1	1	2	2
rye flour	0	0	0	1	1	1	1
self-rising flour	76	302	403	604	805	906	1208
whole-wheat flour	0	1	1	2	3	3	4
DAIRY							
buttermilk	20	78	104	156	208	234	312
evaporated milk	17	63	84	126	168	189	252
skim milk	8	31	42	63	83	94	125
2% fat milk	8	30	40	60	80	90	120
whole milk	8	30	40	60	80	90	120
SWEETS							
brown sugar	3	13	17	26	35	39	52
chocolate chips	2	8	11	16	21	24	32
coconut, fresh	1	4	5	8	11	12	16
coconut, sweet	14	55	73	110	146	164	219
corn syrup	30	120	160	240	320	360	480
honey	1	4	5	8	11	12	16
molasses	8	32	43	64	85	96	128
powdered sugar	0	0	0	0	0	0	0
raisins	3	12	16	24	31	35	47
white sugar	0	0	0	0	0	0	0
FATS							
margarine	141	563	750	1125	1500	1688	2250
margarine, "lite"	131	525	699	1049	1399	1574	2098
margarine, unsalted	2	8	10	15	20	23	30
peanut butter	97	388	518	777	1035	1165	1553
shortening	0	0	0	0	0	0	0

Sodium (mg) in Foods Used in Baking *continued*

Food	1 Tbsp	¼ Cup	⅓ Cup	½ Cup	⅔ Cup	¾ Cup	1 Cup
vegetable oil	1	6	7	11	15	17	22
walnuts	0	0	0	0	0	0	0

MISCELLANEOUS	¼ tsp	½ tsp	1 tsp	1 tbsp			
baking powder	110	219	438	1314			
baking soda	205	411	821	2463			
cocoa powder	0	0	1	3			
salt	541	1082	2164	6491			
salt, "lite"	225	550	1100	3300			
yeast	0	0	0	0			

EGGS	1	2	3	4	5		
egg white	61	122	182	244	304		
egg yolk	8	16	24	32	40		
whole egg	69	138	206	276	344		

Potassium (mg) in Foods Used in Baking

Food	1 Tbsp	¼ Cup	⅓ Cup	½ Cup	⅔ Cup	¾ Cup	1 Cup
GRAIN							
all-purpose flour	7	27	35	53	71	80	106
cake flour	6	24	31	47	63	71	95
cornmeal	18	72	96	144	192	216	288
oatmeal	19	74	99	148	197	222	296
rye flour	14	57	76	114	151	170	227
self-rising flour	6	25	34	51	67	76	101
whole-wheat flour	28	111	148	222	296	333	444
DAIRY							
buttermilk	21	84	112	168	224	252	336
evaporated milk	53	211	280	422	564	634	845
skim milk	22	87	116	174	232	261	348
2% fat milk	23	93	124	186	247	278	371
whole milk	22	87	115	173	231	260	346
SWEETS							
brown sugar	32	129	172	258	343	386	515
chocolate chips	32	126	168	252	336	378	504
coconut, fresh	47	187	249	373	497	560	746
coconut, sweet	17	68	91	137	182	205	273
corn syrup	65	261	348	522	695	782	1043
honey	10	41	54	82	109	122	163
molasses	300	1200	1600	2400	3200	3600	4800
powdered sugar	0	0	0	0	0	0	0
raisins	68	272	363	544	725	816	1088
white sugar	0	0	0	0	0	0	0
FATS							
margarine	3	13	17	26	35	39	52
margarine, "lite"	3	13	17	26	35	39	52
margarine, unsalted	3	13	17	26	35	39	52
peanut butter	107	429	572	858	1143	1286	1715
shortening	0	0	0	0	0	0	0

Potassium (mg) in Foods Used in Baking *continued*

Food	1 Tbsp	¼ Cup	⅓ Cup	½ Cup	⅔ Cup	¾ Cup	1 Cup
vegetable oil	0	0	0	0	0	0	0
walnuts	36	145	193	290	387	435	580

MISCELLANEOUS	¼ tsp	½ tsp	1 tsp	1 tbsp
baking powder	0	0	1	3
baking soda	0	0	0	0
cocoa powder	0	0	1	3
salt	0	0	0	0
salt, "lite"	375	750	1500	4500
yeast	13	27	53	160

EGGS	1	2	3	4	5
egg white	50	100	150	200	250
egg yolk	15	30	45	60	75
whole egg	65	130	195	260	325

Seasoning Alternatives for Foods

Applesauce	cinnamon
Bread	allspice, garlic, poppy seeds
Cabbage	caraway seeds
Cakes	allspice, cinnamon, cloves, ginger, lemon, nutmeg, vanilla extract
Cauliflower	nutmeg
Cheese	mustard
Chicken	basil, bay leaf, curry powder, lemon, sage, tarragon, thyme
Chocolate milk	vanilla extract
Clam chowder	curry powder
Coffee	cinnamon
Cookies	anise, cinnamon, cloves, ginger, nutmeg, poppy seeds, vanilla extract
Corn	chili powder, paprika
Cottage cheese	chives
Cranberry juice	cloves
Cream cheese	chives
Croutons	garlic
Cucumbers	dill, vinegar
Doughnuts	mace
Dressing	marjoram, sage
Eggnog	nutmeg
Eggs	cayenne pepper, chili powder, curry powder, pepper
Eggs, deviled	mustard
Egg salad	oregano
Fish	allspice, basil, cayenne pepper, curry powder, garlic, lemon, oregano, paprika, parsley, tarragon, vinegar
Fish chowder	curry powder
French dressing	curry powder
Fruit	cinnamon, ginger
Fruit, stewed	cinnamon sticks

Seasoning Alternatives for Foods *continued*

Garnish	chervil, fennel, lemon, mint, parsley
Gravy	allspice, mustard
Green beans	mint, oregano
Ham	cloves, mustard
Hamburger	celery seeds, mustard
Indian dishes	turmeric
Irish stew	celery seeds
Italian dishes	garlic, onion, oregano, parsley, pepper
Lamb	mint
Lasagna	garlic
Liver	caraway seeds
Meat	allspice, bell pepper, cayenne pepper, curry powder, onion, parsley, pepper, vinegar
Mexican dishes	chili powder, paprika, pepper
Mincemeat	cinnamon
Noodles	dill, parsley
Omelet	chives
Oriental dishes	ginger
Oysters	chili powder, mace
Pears	ginger, cinnamon
Pickling	cinnamon sticks, cloves, coriander
Pies	allspice, cinnamon, cloves
Pizza	garlic
Popcorn	garlic powder
Pork	basil, caraway seeds, tarragon
Potato salad	celery seeds
Pound cake	mace
Puddings	allspice, cloves, ginger, nutmeg, vanilla extract
Pumpkin pie	allspice, cloves, ginger
Rice	parsley, turmeric
Roast beef	basil
Rolls	poppy seeds
Rye bread	caraway seeds

Seasoning Alternatives for Foods *continued*

Salad	bell pepper, chervil, chives, onion, parsley, rosemary, sorrel, vinegar
Salad dressing	celery seeds, mustard, poppy seeds
Sauces	cayenne pepper, coriander, fennel, rosemary
Seafood	chili powder, lemon, paprika
Soup	bay leaf, chervil, savory, sorrel
Spaghetti sauce	garlic
Spinach	nutmeg, oregano
Steak	tarragon
Stew	bay leaf, cloves, marjoram, rosemary, savory
Tea	cloves, lemon, mint
Tomatoes	celery seeds, curry powder, oregano
Tomato soup	celery seeds
Turkey	basil, bay leaf, marjoram, sage, savory, thyme
Vegetables	basil, bell pepper, chives, dill, lemon, onion, parsley, pepper, savory, sorrel
Vegetable soup	onion, thyme

Uses for Various Seasonings

Allspice	bread, cakes, pies, puddings, relish
Allspice, whole	fish, gravy, meat
Anise	cookies
Basil	chicken, fish, pork, roast beef, turkey, vegetables
Bay leaf	chicken, soup, stew, turkey
Bell pepper	meat, salad, vegetables
Caraway seeds	cabbage, liver, pork, rye bread
Cayenne pepper	eggs, fish, meat, sauces
Celery seeds	hamburger, Irish stew, potato salad, salad dressing, tomatoes, tomato soup
Chervil	garnish, salad, soup
Chili powder	corn, eggs, Mexican dishes, oysters, seafood
Chives	cottage cheese, cream cheese, omelet, salad, vegetables
Cinnamon	applesauce, cakes, coffee, cookies, fruit, mincemeat, pears, pumpkin pie
Cinnamon sticks	pickling, stewed fruit
Cloves	cakes, cookies, cranberry juice, pies, puddings, stew
Cloves, whole	ham, pickling, tea
Coriander	pickling, sauces
Curry powder	chicken, clam chowder, eggs, fish, fish chowder, French dressing, meat, tomatoes
Dill	cucumbers, noodles, vegetables
Fennel	garnish, sauces
Garlic	bread, croutons, fish, Italian dishes, lasagna, pizza, popcorn, spaghetti sauce
Ginger	cakes, cookies, fruit, Oriental dishes, pears, puddings, pumpkin pie
Lemon	cakes, chicken, fish, garnish, seafood, tea, vegetables
Mace	doughnuts, fish, oyster stew, pound cake
Marjoram	dressing, stew, turkey
Mint	garnish, green beans, lamb, tea

Uses for Various Seasonings *continued*

Mustard	cheese, deviled eggs, frankfurter, gravy, ham, hamburger, salad dressing
Nutmeg	cakes, cauliflower, cookies, eggnog, puddings, spinach
Onion	Italian dishes, meat, vegetables, vegetable soup
Oregano	egg salad, fish, green beans, Italian dishes, spinach, tomatoes
Paprika	corn, fish, Mexican dishes, seafood
Parsley	fish, garnish, Italian dishes, meat, noodles, rice, salad, vegetables
Pepper	eggs, Italian dishes, meat, Mexican dishes, vegetables
Poppy seeds	bread, cookies, rolls, salad dressing
Rosemary	salad, sauces, stew
Sage	chicken, dressing, turkey
Savory	soup, stew, turkey, vegetables
Sorrel	salad, soup, vegetables
Tarragon	chicken, fish, pork, steak
Turmeric	Indian dishes
Vanilla extract	cakes, chocolate milk, cookies, puddings
Vinegar	cucumbers, fish, meat, salad

Fast Foods

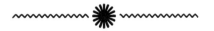

F ast foods are a way of life. Today, it is common for both husband and wife to work. Eating out becomes affordable and convenient. Americans spend $50 billion each year on fast foods. Most Americans purchase a fast-food meal a couple of times each week.

As you study the following tables, you will learn that fast foods can be very high in sodium and fat. A typical cheeseburger and a small order of French fries contain 1 gram of sodium and 26 grams of fat. Forty to 50 percent of the calories comes from fat.

Now that you are making healthy food decisions, you may wonder if it is possible to eat out without blowing your diet. Let the following tables help you to make food decisions for health.

Burger King

Food	HF	Cals	Na+	K+	Fat	% Fat
BEVERAGES:						
Diet Pepsi	0	4	10	32	0	0
orange juice	−9	84	2	348	0	0
milk, 2% low fat	−4*	125	122	377	5	36
milk, whole	−4*	157	119	368	9	52
Pepsi Cola, regular	0	160	10	13	0	0
BREAKFAST:						
Croissan'wich, plain	24*	295	637	149	19	58
w. bacon	29*	352	762	182	24	61
w. ham	36*	328	987	256	20	55
w. sausage	38*	529	1043	285	41	70
egg platter	23*	462	808	487	30	58
w. bacon	29*	532	975	532	36	61
w. sausage	37*	696	1213	623	52	67
French toast sticks	18*	493	498	126	29	53
Great Danish	10*	504	288	116	36	64
BURGER:						
bacon dbl. cheeseburger	22*	519	728	363	31	54
cheeseburger	22*	323	651	247	15	42
hamburger	16*	284	509	235	12	38
Whopper	24*	616	880	545	36	53
Whopper w. cheese	36*	703	1164	568	43	55
Whopper Jr.	14*	333	486	275	17	46
Whopper Jr. w. cheese	20*	372	628	287	20	48
NOT A BURGER:						
chicken sandwich	52*	688	1423	375	40	52
chicken tenders	23*	210	636	200	10	43
ham & cheese sandwich	56*	479	1534	419	23	43
Whaler fish sandwich	16*	499	592	369	27	49
SIDE ORDERS:						
French fries	−2*	225	160	360	13	52
onion rings	25*	272	665	173	16	53

*fat = 20 or more percent of calories

Burger King *continued*

Food	HF	Cals	Na+	K+	Fat	% Fat
salad, plain	−9	28	23	382	0	0
w. blue cheese	4*	184	332	400	16	78
w. house dressing	2*	161	292	402	13	73
w. low-calorie Italian	10	36	449	388	0	0
w. 1000 Island dressing	1*	152	251	404	12	71
DESSERTS:						
apple pie	15*	296	412	122	12	36
chocolate shake	−6*	324	202	567	12	33
vanilla shake	−4*	322	205	505	10	28

*fat = 20 or more percent of calories

Hardee's

Food	HF	Cals	Na	K	Fat	% Fat
BEVERAGES:						
Coke, regular	0	160	10	13	0	0
Diet Coke	0	4	10	32	0	0
milk, 2% low fat	−4*	125	122	377	5	36
milk, whole	−4*	157	119	368	9	52
orange juice	−9	84	2	348	0	0
BURGER:						
bacon cheeseburger	28*	556	888	431	33	53
Big Deluxe	28*	503	903	426	29	52
big roast beef	47*	440	1323	411	22	44
cheeseburger	31*	309	825	202	13	37
hamburger	22*	276	589	148	15	50
¼-pound hamburger	39*	511	1112	360	28	50
roast beef	30*	312	826	241	12	36
NOT A BURGER:						
chicken fillet	7*	510	360	334	26	46
fish fillet	32*	469	1013	465	20	39
ham 'n' cheese	38*	375	1067	317	15	36
hot dog	30*	346	768	120	22	57
turkey club sandwich	40*	426	1185	444	22	47
SIDE ORDERS:						
chef salad	12*	277	517	414	16	52
French fries	−2*	239	180	401	13	49
side salad	−1	21	42	101	0	4
DESSERTS:						
apple turnover	3*	282	216	270	14	44
big cookie	10*	278	258	64	15	50
milkshake	−1	391	241	433	10	24

*fat = 20 or more percent of calories

McDonald's

Food	HF	Cals	Na	K	Fat	% Fat
BREAKFAST:						
Egg McMuffin	34*	331	885	168	15	40
English muffin	12*	185	318	71	5	26
hash brown potato	8*	124	325	247	7	51
hotcakes, butter & syrup	42	499	1070	187	10	19
pork sausage	24*	205	615	127	19	82
scrambled eggs	6*	180	205	135	13	65
BURGER:						
Big Mac	38*	566	1010	237	34	54
cheeseburger	29*	306	767	156	14	41
hamburger	19*	254	520	142	10	35
McDLT	36*	680	1030	330	44	58
Quarter Pounder	24*	421	735	322	22	46
Quarter Pounder w. cheese	45*	522	1236	341	31	53
NOT A BURGER:						
filet-o-fish	30*	431	781	150	25	52
SIDE ORDERS:						
French fries, regular	−10*	218	109	564	12	47
DESSERTS:						
apple pie	16*	252	398	39	14	51
caramel sundae	0*	328	195	338	10	27
cherry pie	18*	258	427	35	14	47
chocolate shake	−2	381	300	580	9	21
hot fudge sundae	−3*	309	175	410	11	31
ice cream cone	−1*	185	109	221	5	25
McDonald's cookie	14*	308	358	52	11	32
strawberry shake	−2	363	207	423	9	22
strawberry sundae	−3*	288	96	290	9	27
vanilla shake	−2	351	201	422	8	22

*fat = 20 or more percent of calories

Pizza

Food	HF	Cals	Na	K	Fat	% Fat
½ of 10-in pizza						
thick crust	40	457	1132	368	6	12
thin crust	41*	355	1116	285	10	25
½ of 12-in pizza						
regular crust	46	650	1347	474	12	17

*fat = 20 or more percent of calories

Taco Bell

Food	HF	Cals	Na	K	Fat	% Fat
BURRITO						
bean burrito	29*	363	922	428	11	27
beef burrito	35*	396	994	313	17	39
burrito supreme	30*	422	952	437	19	40
combo burrito	35*	379	958	370	14	33
dbl. beef supreme	35*	461	1054	434	23	45
supreme platter	58*	768	1920	991	37	42
MISCELLANEOUS:						
Bell beefer	30*	312	855	298	13	38
Cinnamon Crispas	4*	263	1222	36	16	54
enchirito	44*	382	1260	423	20	47
nachos	14*	353	423	159	19	49
nachos Bellgrande	38*	718	1312	763	41	51
pintos & cheese	22*	197	733	384	9	43
Pizzazz Pizza	48*	712	1364	449	48	61
TACO:						
soft taco	18*	225	516	178	9	45
taco	8*	182	273	159	11	54
taco Bellgrande	12*	345	470	334	22	56
taco light	17*	407	575	316	29	64
TACO PLATTER:						
Bellgrande	61*	1001	1962	946	51	46
light	66*	1062	2068	923	58	49
TACO SALAD:						
plain	45*	955	1741	1212	62	59
without beans	36*	824	1345	885	57	62
without shell	36*	530	1500	1141	32	55
w. ranch dressing	61*	1210	2047	1110	91	68
TOSTADA:						
beefy tostada	20*	313	706	406	19	53
tostada	19*	247	670	401	11	41

*fat = 20 or more percent of calories

Taco Bell *continued*

Food	HF	Cals	Na	K	Fat	% Fat
SEAFOOD SALAD:						
plain	55*	928	1567	501	70	68
no dressing	28*	656	917	450	41	57
no shell	20*	230	677	379	11	45

*fat = 20 or more percent of calories

Wendy's

Food	HF	Cals	Na	K	Fat	% Fat
BREAKFAST:						
bacon	18*	112	445	65	10	80
breakfast sandwich	30*	371	770	155	19	46
French toast	33*	395	850	175	19	43
home fries	17*	362	745	615	22	55
omelet						
w. mushroom & onion	4*	219	200	190	15	62
w. ham & cheese	13*	249	405	180	17	61
w. ham, cheese, & mushroom	20*	289	570	190	21	65
sausage	15*	200	410	125	18	81
scrambled eggs	4*	192	160	130	12	56
toast w. margarine	16*	245	410	80	9	33
BURGER:						
¼ lb, bacon & cheese	29*	460	860	330	28	55
¼ lb, wheat bun	5*	333	290	310	17	46
¼ lb, white bun	11*	354	410	275	18	46
½ lb, white bun	13*	566	575	485	34	54
NOT A BURGER:						
chicken, wheat bun	14*	314	500	320	10	29
chili, 8 oz	32*	260	1070	565	8	28
taco salad	28*	398	1100	790	18	41
BAKED POTATO:						
plain	−32	250	60	1360	2	7
w. bacon & cheese	16*	574	1180	1380	30	47
w. broccoli & cheese	−21*	493	430	1550	25	46
w. chili & cheese	−14*	520	610	1590	20	35
w. cheese	−16*	594	450	1380	34	52
w. sour cream	−6*	452	230	1420	24	48
SIDE ORDERS:						
French fries	−12*	282	95	635	14	45
side salad	15*	106	540	320	6	51

*fat = 20 or more percent of calories

Wendy's *continued*

Food	HF	Cals	Na	K	Fat	% Fat
SALAD DRESSINGS *(1 oz)*:						
blue cheese	7*	138	170	20	14	91
celery seed	6*	146	139	11	13	79
golden Italian	22*	100	520	20	8	72
1000 Island	9*	146	230	30	14	86
ranch	13*	170	310	20	18	95
red French	10*	134	260	40	10	67
REDUCED CALORIE:						
bacon & tomato	13*	92	320	50	8	78
creamy cucumber	12*	110	280	20	10	82
1000 Island	10*	92	250	40	8	78
Italian	15*	56	360	20	4	64
wine vinegar	0	4	10	20	0	0
DESSERT:						
Frosty	−5*	394	220	585	14	32

*fat = 20 or more percent of calories

Are We Realistic?

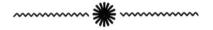

A sk someone else to do it. It's so easy. Shift the responsibility of making the food decision to a nutritionist, physician, nurse, or family member. Health care providers have more experience. They are interested. Is this true? Yes. Does it work? No. My job is to provide the tools so you can develop food skills and achieve health goals.

Set goals that offer benefits. The benefits will motivate you to continue to achieve your health goals over time. Today, you may choose to select foods for health. That's a general decision. This morning, you may choose to eat sausage. That's a single, specific decision related to time. It's up to me, as a nutritionist, to provide information so you can achieve the big decision through the sum of many specific small food-for-health decisions. The process must be realistic and safe.

A pound of body fat is equal to 3,500 calories. To set realistic goals, consult the 1983 Metropolitan Life Tables for optimal weights in the chapter on risk factors. If you weigh within ten pounds of the optimal weight for your height, a loss of one pound per week is realistic. If you weigh thirty or more pounds above optimal weight, a loss of two to three pounds per week is realistic. The rate of weight loss will decrease one or two pounds per week as you approach optimal weight.

How much time will it take to reach your goal? It may take a year to lose fifty pounds! That may seem like a very long time. Think of the impatient child who can't wait till Christmas. Sometimes you have to wait till Christmas. Keep on track.

Intent starts but does not equal reality. Our lives are filled with plenty of good intentions. Selecting foods for health requires accepting the responsibility for making one hundred daily food decisions. These decisions include choosing twenty to thirty foods and beverages, food preparation, and food portion, as well as many decisions to not consume specific foods that are easily available. We must make decisions actively. If we are passive, nothing will change.

Set specific goals. General goals tend to foster a delayed recognition of achievement. All of us want to be "better" people. It sounds like a "good" idea to be a "better" person. However, being a "better" person means nothing until you can measure it. The measure of many food decisions can be found on the bathroom scales. You can stand on the scales and know if you're achieving your goal. However, it takes time to see the difference on the scales. Remember that achieving the general goal is the sum of achieving many smaller specific goals.

However, general goals by themselves lead to laziness. A general goal is not sufficiently specific to monitor achievement. The general goal to lose twenty pounds without spelling out the details is very hard to achieve. A plan with steps works. Consider decisions you make throughout the day.

The following list is just an example of some of the individual small goals you can set for the day. Set your own goals. Be responsible. Be sensitive to your needs and personality.

1. Eat a balanced breakfast.
2. Use a sugar substitute in coffee.
3. Park the car two blocks from work.
4. Do not eat the doughnut that someone so thoughtfully brought to work.
5. Decrease the dressing on the salad at lunch.
6. Eat half the French fries you would normally eat.
7. Substitute a diet soda for a regular soda this afternoon.
8. Eat fruit for a snack rather than a candy bar.
9. Take the opportunity to walk up some steps.
10. Get rid of that bag of potato chips.
11. Bake the meat for dinner tonight.
12. Have a glass of skim milk when you feel hungry.
13. Have a baked potato with yogurt and chives rather than sour cream and butter.
14. Walk two miles to earn an ice cream (soft ice milk) cone without feeling guilty.
15. Be happy and recognize your effort!
16. Make your list of small goals!

Try using worksheets for setting realistic daily goals related to your weight over time.

Expectations from changing the food-decision process leading to weight normalization should be realistic. The rate of weight loss has already been discussed. Expectations as to changes in personality, social life, and happiness are separate issues. It is hoped that through weight normalization you will obtain good health. Self-confidence, pride, and happiness may result from good health.

Attitudes about what you should or should not weigh must be realistic. Regardless of how much they weigh, the majority of women in this country generally stand on the scales and say immediately that their weight should be five to ten pounds less. I do this. Be realistic. Be fair to yourself when setting goals for optimal weight.

Keeping Motivated

There will always be times when you don't want to think about what you eat, when you eat, and how much you eat. The details can be very boring. There is so much repetition. "What are we having for supper tonight?" Moms and Dads probably get pretty tired of hearing that question. Accept that the enthusiasm will come and go.

You will reach a point when the decisions are made by automatic pilot. Compare the skill to driving a car. It's a learned process. You may be clumsy when you first begin. It becomes easier and automatic when you have successfully reached your first realistic goal.

Accept that there will be times when it's boring. It's a little like brushing your teeth. You just do it. Maybe you will change brands of toothpaste. Brush from the left to the right versus top to bottom to break the monotony. Brushing your teeth will still be boring. Keep the benefits in mind. It's satisfying to go to the dentist and there are no cavities or drilling required. It is satisfying when you stand on the scales and you don't have to cringe! You will see the benefits of weight normalization. You will be proud!

Some of us are motivated by a scare. When a close friend or a family member of long-term excess weight becomes very sick with an illness that can be related to that excess weight, the message is clear that life is precious. You may become aware of your own vulnerability. All of us are individually responsible for our health. You cannot turn the clock backward. However, today is the first day of the rest of your life!

Consider the following activities to aid you decrease boredom and maintain your enthusiasm for helping yourself.

Keep a food diary of the foods you have chosen not to consume. This will emphasize the many food decisions that you make throughout the day.

Seek new recipes to vary foods you eat. If the recipe is low in fat, it can probably be successfully incorporated into your food pattern.

Sometimes people overeat when they are depressed. If you are feeling down, consider alternative activities that you enjoy. Perhaps going to a movie can lift your spirits. The day will always be brighter with fresh flowers around. Taking a walk often helps because it is clearly a positive step. When you take a walk, you are stating that you care about yourself.

Do not use food as a reward. Think of food as something essential for life. You eat food to supply the body with needed nutrients. Also, healthy food can be used in social situations in a way that is quite enjoyable. Just be sensible and plan ahead.

Find other people who are trying to normalize their body weight. Group support often helps. Perhaps you and your co-workers can start a kitty to which each person contributes a dollar every week. The person who makes the greatest progress toward satisfying his or her health goal wins the kitty for that week.

Change your goals for a week or more. Concentrate on weight reduction during week one and week two. Make it a goal to maintain or not gain weight during week three. This will test your automatic pilot, or the changes you have successfully incorporated into your daily life. Return to weight reduction during week four.

Accept that normalizing body weight is a series of many decisions. The most important single decision is that your food choices will be based on health.

Conversion Factors and Abbreviations

CALORIE SOURCE:

Alc	— alcohol	7 cal/gm
Cal	— calorie(s)	
Cho	— carbohydrate	4 cal/gm
Fat	— fat	9 cal/gm
Pro	— protein	4 cal/gm

DISTANCE:

cm	— centimeter(s)	1 cm	= 0.4 in
in	— inch(es)	1 in	= 2.54 cm
m	— meter	1 m	= 1.09 yd
mm	— millimeter(s)	1 mm	= 0.001 m
yd	— yard	1 yd	= 0.91 m

MINERALS:

Ca	— calcium	Mn	= manganese
Cu	— copper	Na	= sodium
Fe	— iron	O	= oxygen
Hg	— mercury	P	= phosphorus
I	— iodine	S	= sulfur
K	— potassium	Zn	= zinc
Mg	— magnesium		

MISCELLANEOUS:

mmHg — millimeters of mercury
mph — miles per hour
mEq — milliequivalent   1 mEq Na = 23 mg Na
                             1 mEq K = 39 mg K

TIME:

hr — hour(s)
min — minute(s)
yr — year(s)

WEIGHT:

gm — gram(s)   1 oz = 30 gm
kg — kilogram(s)   1 kg = 2.2 lb
lb — pound(s)   1 lb = 0.454 kg
mg — milligram(s)   1 gm = 1000 mg
oz — ounce(s)   1 lb = 16 oz

BEE — basal energy expenditure
BMI — body mass index
HDL — high-density lipoprotein
HF   — Heart Factor
IBW — ideal body weight
LDL — low-density lipoprotein
SF   — salt-free
VLDL — very-low-density lipoprotein

Index

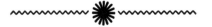